M000252114

Cases in Food Service and Clinical Nutrition Management

Edited by:

Amy Allen-Chabot, Ph.D., R.D.
Associate Professor
Anne Arundel Community College

Ken Jarvis, MBA
Associate Professor
Anne Arundel Community College

Robert M. O'Halloran, Ph.D.
Professor & Director
Kemmons Wilson School of Hospitality & Resort Management
University of Memphis

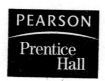

PEARSON
Prentice
Hall

Upper Saddle River, New Jersey 07458

Library of Congress Cataloging-in-Publication Data
Cases in food service and clinical nutrition management/edited by Amy Allen-Chabot,
  Ken Jarvis, Robert M. O'Halloran.
    p. cm.
   Includes biographical references.
   ISBN 0-13-111464-6 (pbk.)
    1. Hospitals—Food service—Case studies. 2. Diet therapy—Case studies. I.
Allen-Chabot, Amy. II. Jarvis, Ken, III. O'Halloran, Robert M.

RA975.5.D5C37 2006
642'.56—dc22

2004061738

Executive Editor: Vernon R. Anthony
Editorial Assistant: Beth Dyke
Executive Marketing Manager: Ryan DeGrote
Senior Marketing Coordinator: Elizabeth Farrell
Director of Manufacturing & Production: Bruce Johnson
Managing Editor: Mary Carnis
Production Liaison: Janice Stangel
Production Editor: Ann Mohan, WordCrafters Editorial Services, Inc.
Manufacturing Manager: Ilene Sanford
Manufacturing Buyer: Cathleen Petersen
Marketing Assistant: Les Roberts
Creative Director: Cheryl Asherman
Senior Design Coordinator: Miguel Ortiz
Cover Design: Amy Rosen
Cover Image: Getty Images/Comstock Images
Interior Design and Composition: Pine Tree Composition, Inc.
Printer/Binder: Courier Stoughton

Copyright 2006 by Pearson Education, Inc., Upper Saddle River, New Jersey, 07458. Pearson Prentice
Hall. All rights reserved. Printed in the United States of America. This publication is protected by Copyright
and permission should be obtained from the publisher prior to any prohibited reproduction, storage in a
retrieval system, or transmission in any form or by any means, electronic, mechanical, photocopying, recording, or likewise. For information regarding permission(s), write to: Rights and Permissions Department.

Pearson Prentice Hall™ is a trademark of Pearson Education, Inc.
Pearson® is a registered trademark of Pearson plc
Prentice Hall® is a registered trademark of Pearson Education, Inc.

Pearson Education LTD.
Pearson Education Singapore, Pte. Ltd.
Pearson Education, Canada, Ltd.
Pearson Education–Japan
Pearson Education Australia PTY, Limited
Pearson Education North Asia Ltd.
Pearson Educación de Mexico, S.A. de C.V.
Pearson Education Malaysia, Pte. Ltd.

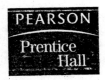

10 9 8 7 6 5 4 3
ISBN 0-13-111464-6

This book is dedicated to
Suzanne R. Curtis, Ph.D., R.D.,
a beloved friend and valued contributor
to the field of food service and dietetics.

Contents

Cases in Management of Food Services

Cases in Nutrition Management

Cases in Financial Management

Introduction

This text provides learning opportunities in food service and clinical nutrition management through the use of case studies. By studying these cases, you can build on your knowledge, comprehend complex situations, apply theory, analyze situations, create solutions, and evaluate and select outcomes. In the process, you will hone your decision-making skills.

The significance of case studies as learning tools is that there can be many solutions justified by different points of view given similar data and information. Some of the cases in this text provide extensive data; others require assumptions, speculation, and creativity in the decision-making process. It is important to note that it is the thinking and decision-making processes you use that ultimately enhance your learning.

As you read these cases, use the following framework as a guide.

Case Framework for Students

1. *Read the case.*
2. *Identify the relevant content.*
3. *Identify the problem.* Differentiate between symptoms and problems. Is the problem in marketing, human resources, finance, or some other area?
4. *Identify the relevant facts.* Which facts are most important for decision making?
5. *Identify assumptions you may be making.*

6. *Generate plausible alternatives for the case.* Should you do nothing? Spend a lot of money to fix the problems? Since neither of these alternatives is typically an acceptable solution, you need to formulate viable alternatives.

7. *Make a decision based on your alternatives.* Decision making requires a balance of information and the ability to evaluate data for their importance. You also need to understand whether the alternatives you have developed are workable. Therefore, a discussion with a faculty member on the decision-making process might be appropriate. A sample decision-making process follows.

Sample Decision-Making Process

1. *Identify the issue.* Is it a well-structured or ill-structured problem? Does it have one solution?

2. *Collect facts and evidence.* What are the facts? Differentiate fact from opinion. Which decision-making tools are needed?

3. *Make judgments and decide alternative results.* Collect new facts. What are the possible outcomes of different judgments?

4. *Identify what role, if any, an individual's experience in the workplace plays in the decision.* Weigh experience in similar situations.

5. *Evaluate the evidence.* Ask the right questions. Decide what criteria are being used to weigh the evidence. Which pieces of evidence will you use to make your decision?

6. *Reach a conclusion (judgment).*

It is critical to identify the type of problem the individuals are facing in a case. Is there one right answer? Next, identify the facts and information that are most relevant to the decision-making process. Not all facts in a case will have the same importance. You will decide which evidence or information is most important. The identification of the main issue or problem is a key goal of the case method.

Many cases will be ill structured; others may have a preferred solution. Cases may have different orientations. The key issue for some might be marketing; for others it might be communication; while still others might involve organizational behavior, decision making, or supervision. Each case has its own direction, and it should be the facts of that case that determine the direction of the outcome. In the analysis stage of the case process, the reader must be able to identify the most important aspects of the situation given the facts of the case, the problem, and the probable outcome.

An individual's personal experiences and expertise are also involved in this process. Each person is likely to look at the facts of a case differently. Expert opinion can also be helpful in characterizing a situation. If facts in a case indicate that the president of a company or a consultant provided input, then their credibility can influence your decision.

The food service and clinical nutrition management arena is rich with examples and opportunities for learning. The case studies presented in this text provide a broad spectrum of situations, issues, and learning opportunities from which to select.

Acknowledgments

We thank the following reviewers for their valuable feedback on this book:

Kathleen M. O'Brien, Buffalo State College
Julie Lengfelder, Bowling Green State University

We would also like to express our thanks to the following authors who contributed case studies included in this book:

Melissa Altman-Traub, M.S., R.D.
Lois Black, R.D., L.D./N
Julie J. Davis, M.S., R.D., L.D.
Gina Hinch, D.T.R.
Linda R. Hofmeister, M.M., R.D., L.D., F.A.D.A., C.H.E.
Marcia Johnson, R.D., C.D.
Theresa Kevak, M.S., R.D., L.D./N
Amy Knoblock-Hahn, M.S., R.D., L.D.
Susan Kosharek, M.S., R.D., L.D.
Teresa T. Marcus, M.S., R.D., L.D./N
Nancy L. Matyas, R.D., L.D.
Laura McKnight, M.P.H., R.D., L.D.
Phyllis Fatzinger McShane, M.S., R.D., L.D.
Kathleen Meyer, R.D., L.D.
Jan Patenaude, R.D.
Naveena Reddy, M.S., R.D., L.D.
Joanne Robinett, M.S., SFNS
Nell E. Robinson, M.S., R.D. L.D./N

Amy Allen-Chabot
Ken Jarvis
Robert M. O'Halloran

Cases in Menu Management

THE HEART OF THE MATTER: THE MENU

INITIATING SUCCESSFUL CHANGE IN THE HEALTHCARE WORK ENVIRONMENT

PATIENT WITH SPECIAL NEEDS

MENU EXTENSIONS IN A HOSPITAL GRILL AND SNACK BAR

HOSPITAL FOOD SERVICE MENU FOR EMERGENCY CONDITIONS

The Heart of the Matter

The Menu

Objectives

At the completion of this case study, students should be able to:

1. Examine the main elements of a menu: cost, production, customer satisfaction (including special needs), and equipment.
2. Recognize the menu as a malleable and essential tool in the successful operation.
3. Underscore the advantages of utilizing a holistic, collaborative approach; available software for nutritional analysis and recipe extension; and dietitians and chefs to save time and increase acceptance by staff and clients.

Case Narrative

Part One

Steffany, Gina, and Thomas eagerly anticipated their latest assignment from their employer. They had three months to plan a new menu, evaluate it for special nutritional needs and adequacy, get recipes in finished form, and get the entire package accepted by their staff of 100. The site was a 600-bed hospital in the lower Midwest. Known for its good food, the hospital's food service customer satisfaction had been taking a nosedive of late. All three agreed that there were a few food quality inconsistencies, but that the root of the problem was related to customer perception. Over and over they heard the patients say that even though the menu offered five entrée choices per meal daily, it was the same five day after day, and so there was no perception of variety or choice.

3

Gina, the production manager, was in charge of a staff that had good cooking skills and was accustomed to preparing large amounts of food. Currently they produced food for an adult daycare center, two childcare buildings, the patient tray line, a huge employee cafeteria, and two outlying clinics. They accomplished this while having to share limited equipment with the catering staff. The present cafeteria menu was an eight-week cycle menu that tried to offer heart healthy items along with meat and potato favorites. Gina suspected that the dietitians, especially Thomas, wanted to make every item heart healthy. They just didn't seem concerned that about 85 percent of total sales were comfort foods and that meat and potatoes were a vast regional favorite. Food waste was less than 5 percent, which was great for such a large kitchen, and the tray line and production crew got handwritten notes regularly from patients who loved the food. To improve customer (patient) satisfaction, six of the hardest-to-please units had recently begun room service, and it was going very well. Gina knew some units would never be on room service and was concerned about keeping the quality of food for all the other customers good while introducing new menus and food items.

Thomas was an excellent dietitian who viewed the production staff (including Gina) as cantankerous, not at all customer oriented, and blissfully ignorant about nutritional concerns. Thomas also had many allergy problems, was a vegetarian, and was outspoken about the inadequacy of the menus for those two concerns. Secretly, he hoped to write a menu to address this and felt that it would benefit the general population to eat foods from this regimen.

Steffany dreaded the whole process in a way. She had been cooking here for twenty years and had seen many menus come and go. Very patient-satisfaction oriented, Steffany knew there was room for improvement. She also knew that any change would be painful for the crew, since most of them hated change of any sort. There had been a lot of budgetary cutbacks recently, so she hoped that the workload would not be too unreasonable for the existing staff and that the food quality would not suffer. Wondering whether she would have to spend all of the planning time mediating between Gina and Thomas, Steffany was anxious about proceeding with the project.

Questions

1. Who should be involved in the process of writing a new menu?
2. How might the team proceed at this point in getting the necessary input from the key people identified in Question 1?

Part Two

The process began with two discussions about food items. Favorite food items of past and present and some new ones were suggested, and items to be removed were scratched off the list. From these discussions attended by dietitians, production staff, and tray line crew, a list of regular diet items was identified. Dietitians then took the list and wrote the menus, extending the regular menu to all the special diet needs. Thomas took advantage of the situation to write a much-needed vegetarian menu and to instill as many low-fat, vegetarian items as he could. He also added recipes.

Gina took the menu and evaluated it for food cost per patient meal, ingredient availability, and appropriateness of recipes to be extended for modified diets. Because the same kitchen produced different menus for different customers at the same time, availability of equipment and staff had to be considered. Gina broke the menu down in terms of workload per station (e.g., vegetables, ovens, salads), and dovetailed it to see that everyone could handle the new expectations. Steffany had the assignment of preparing some of the unfamiliar recipes to see whether they held up to needed time and temperature guidelines and whether the presentation at point of service was desirable. Tray line workers began drafting steam table diagrams to be sure they could accommodate all the food items in a timely fashion.

This done, the group got together to discuss their findings. The biggest disagreement came over the acceptance of "healthy, vegetarian, heart healthy" foods and preparation techniques versus "great tasting food." With Steffany's encouragement, Thomas and Gina finally agreed that a moderate approach to healthy food, prepared in a variety of methods, was most likely to satisfy the most customers. Thomas was able to keep his vegetarian menu, but it was specific to vegetarians. With the assistance of *Food Processor* software, nutritional analyses were completed and recipes extended.

The end product was a seven-day-cycle menu that was cost efficient and dovetailed nicely with the existing cafeteria and daycare menus. The staff in all the production areas were given recipes and time to practice preparation, holding, and dipping to achieve consistent quality. With batch cooking, *C-Bord* patient menu software, and careful observation of time and temperature windows, waste was expected to improve slightly over the current 5 percent. All three individuals were satisfied with the final product. They had also received an unexpected benefit: The collaboration of three different perspectives resulted in a better product for the patient, and a sense of teamwork and improved morale for the staff.

Questions

1. What effect do personal tastes or professional perspectives have on menu writing?
2. At what point is it important to assess client needs and expectations?
3. For a successful result, how would you prioritize food cost, production, presentation, and customer satisfaction?
4. Would success be defined differently for different types of facilities (e.g. restaurant versus institutional, or even cafeteria versus in-patient dietary within the same institution)?

Initiating Successful Change in the Healthcare Work Environment

Objectives

At the completion of this case study, students should be able to:

1. Understand that employees often resist change.
2. Be familiar with ways of establishing an atmosphere for positive change.
3. Recognize the value of feedback when assessing change.

Case Narrative

Today, the food service department is constantly challenged with providing excellent service while containing cost. José, the food service director at a medium-sized hospital, faced this dilemma when he was asked by administration to reduce the labor and food budget for the next fiscal year. Accomplishing this reduction required major changes in the department. To start, he looked at the menu, which dictates costs for food, supplies, and labor. The facility had a seven-day cycle, each day offering three entrées for breakfast. At lunch and dinner patients had a choice of four hot and three cold entrées. Also on the menu were offerings of two salads, four desserts, and three types of bread, with four hot and seven cold beverages. After reviewing the menu, he faced a tough decision regarding what to change. He considered cutting out some of the entrée choices, offering less expensive desserts, and so on. He then needed to determine how labor would be impacted by the change. In other words, would it adequately reduce FTEs (full-time equivalents) while maintaining reasonable customer satisfaction?

Food service management must always be open to new advances in techniques, equipment, and products, and this is achieved through readings and networking.

José found an article on the spoken menu and wondered whether he should try it. The spoken menu concept involves someone from the food service department verbally obtaining menu selections prior to each meal rather than sending up a menu the previous day to be marked by the patient. He visited two hospitals with spoken menus to see exactly how it worked. He was sold by what he saw: A brief menu was reviewed with the patient right before meal service (not the day before), and the menu had fewer selections in each food category.

José and his management team had a meeting and presented the general idea to the staff. The team was enthusiastic about implementing the spoken menu in the department. As the team members described the new system, they saw some blinders go up with some of the older employees. Employees stated such things as "Change again," "Do what you want, we just follow orders," and "Here we go again!!" José spent time going over details and answering questions, but the staff was still upset, showing real concern about how it would affect their jobs.

For the next six months, the team gathered information on menus, staffing, and equipment and made plans for the change.

Restructuring

The first step was to create a new menu. The management team decided to offer a select menu but with fewer items in each category. They also chose to offer soup or fresh fruit as an appetizer and only offer two desserts. The menu would be a seven-day cycle and would be given to patients when they arrived at the hospital; the spoken menu concept would be implemented. To assure a savings in time, José decided that the nutrition representatives would take on this job because they could be trained to take selections and keep them in line with the ordered diet, actually correcting the menu as they took the order. This would eliminate a lot of extra work in the diet office.

Weekly meetings were conducted with groups of employees to review the menu, staffing, equipment, and so on. Management reviewed a plan, and the staff would help finalize details. For example, with regard to equipment, the staff felt they would not have enough room in the mobile refrigeration unit, so the decision was made that backup units could hold the extra items. The meetings did help the staff get comfortable with the change.

Since the food service department was proposing a major change in the traditional hospital food service, a detailed presentation was provided to the nursing staff and the hospital administration. Selling the nursing staff on the system was easy since only two FTEs are used on the line due to the simplified menu, resulting in extra staff being available for passing trays. This freed up nursing from this task. In addition, patient requests were now handled exclusively by the dietary department. Nutrition representatives would simply carry a beeper, and changes would be faxed from the floor to the food service. These were all positive impacts on the nursing staff, so they were positive and expressed this to the administration.

The approach to the administration emphasized the fact that patient food selections would be obtained twenty minutes before actual service for all meals. It was also emphasized that the system allows the department to serve new admissions with their selection. This could potentially reduce FTEs by 1.5 and decrease food cost by 5 percent. The monetary investment was only $5,000 for a steam table, refrigerator, and mobile beverage service cart.

With approval from the administration, the management team ordered the equipment and materials. The given plan was to have key management people work along with the staff as the facility established the new program.

The dietitian worked with the nutrition representatives, and the cooks and cold preparation staff were provided guidance regarding production. The hardest thing for the staff to accept was going from five people to two people on the tray assembly line.

It was a long week, but after each meal, with employee input, the management team would refine the process. Meal rounds were completed, and patients were pleased with the meals and service. Staff were also pleased with the workload and really loved the system.

Questions

1. What two obstacles were in place for the start of the program?
2. What are the identified advantages of the spoken menu system?
3. What are some of the possible disadvantages of the spoken menu?
4. Identify strategies used or not used in this case that can help promote positive change and keep anxiety and complications resulting from the change to a minimum.
5. What is the importance of feedback?

Patient with Special Needs

Objectives

At the completion of this case study, students should be able to:

1. Identify the basic clinical nutrition processes in a hospital setting.
2. Find the resources on the gluten-free diet.
3. Describe how to accommodate the special needs of your client.

Case Narrative

Ms. SR is an 83-year-old female admitted to the hospital with the diagnosis of fever and weakness. Her medical history includes celiac disease, severe anemia, and hypertension. She forgot her dentures at the nursing home where she lives; therefore, mechanical soft is added to her gluten-free diet order. The hospital has very limited choices on the menu for gluten-free diets and the mechanical soft restriction further limits the choices.

Her admitting labs showed serum albumin at 2.8 g/dL, suggesting she was somewhat protein deficient. Her weight is 122 lb. and her height is 5 feet, 5 inches. She reported that at the nursing home, she had fair intake of meals, was able to chew regular meat without dentures, and sometimes took Ensure when not able to eat. She was not sure of her weight change. She complained of her poor appetite; however, when it was offered, she agreed to try Boost Plus, a dietary supplement beverage, three times a day with meals. The staff dietitian found her drinking two to three cans of Boost Plus a day and consuming about 25 percent of her meals.

Ms. SR remained in the hospital for more than a week, and her meal intake gradually dropped to 10 percent or less. When asked about the reason for such poor intake, Ms. SR reported that she continued to have a poor appetite and was tired of eating ground meat and the same food frequently. The dietitian attempted to elicit some food preferences. Unfortunately, due to the mechanical soft, gluten-free diet restrictions, she could not offer much of the food Ms. SR preferred. After a series of tests, she was later diagnosed with cervical cancer. The physician was hesitant to treat the condition aggressively due to the patient's poor nutritional status and frail condition. Her serum albumin level dropped from 2.8 to 1.9 g/dL. Other than Boost Plus; her fluid intake was also dropping. The staff dietitian also found that the patient was unhappy with her situation, which was also contributing to her poor intake of meals. She discussed the situation with the chief clinical dietitian.

Questions

1. What is gluten, and what foods would not be allowed on a gluten-free diet?
2. How can you improve variety in Ms. SR's meals?
3. How can you improve patient intake and subsequently patient satisfaction?
4. Would it be okay for Ms. SR's family to bring food in from home? Why or why not?
5. Dietitians often offer canned supplements such as Boost and Ensure to patients who are not eating well. What are the advantages and drawbacks of this?

Reference

Mahan, L., and S. Escott-Stump. 2000. *Krause's food, nutrition and diet therapy.* 10th ed. Philadelphia: W. B. Saunders.

Menu Extensions in a Hospital Grill and Snack Bar

Objectives

At the completion of this case study, students should be able to:

1. Assess a menu in terms of the ingredients required.
2. Develop new menu items with minimal expansion of food inventory.

Case Narrative

Juanita is the manager of a small grill and snack bar located in a large medical center. The grill has been open for one year, and sales have been moderately good. The menu for the operation is as follows:

Hamburgers
Cheeseburgers
Chili (ground beef, beans, tomatoes, tomato-based sauce)
French fries
Garden salads with assorted single serving dressings
Sodas
Iced tea
Coffee

Condiments and toppings for burgers include

Lettuce
Tomato

Mustard
Mayonnaise
Sour cream (for chili)
Ketchup
Bacon
Relish
Barbeque sauce

Part One

Juanita wants to get some customer feedback so she hands out a customer comment card with each check for one month. The card is five by seven inches and is printed with questions on both sides.

Question

What questions might be appropriate for the customer comment card? Design a small customer comment card for this operation.

Part Two

After one month, Juanita looks at all the cards and tallies the results. She finds that customers feel the food is excellent and the service is very good. The most common comment is that more selection is desired. Juanita ponders this and thinks about her limited storage space. She can add some menu items but would like to avoid adding a lot more food items to the inventory.

Question

Add three new menu items to this menu while adding only two new inventory items.

Part Three

The second most common comment that Juanita got on the comment cards was related to healthier menu items. Patrons stated that they would like some healthier or lower fat and/or lower calorie items on the menu. Again, Juanita wanted to provide customers with the items they desired but did not have the space or desire to add a lot of inventory.

Questions

1. How might you define a healthy menu item? Support your definition.
2. Add two new healthy menu items while keeping new inventory items to a minimum.

Hospital Food Service Menu for Emergency Conditions

Objectives

At the completion of this case study, students should be able to:

1. Identify potential emergency situations or disasters in which an alternative menu may be needed.
2. Construct a three-meal menu that does not need heating but still meets the nutritional needs of the hospital patient.
3. Identify nonperishable items that should be kept on hand at all times for use in the event of an emergency. Ideally, most of the items are foods that are normally in the kitchen's inventory.

Case Narrative

Some electrical lines in the neighborhood where Glen Maple Hospital is located are downed at 5:00 A.M. due to a heavy rainstorm. Donna, the opening supervisor, is informed of the problem as she enters the building at 6:00 A.M. The breakfast tray line for the patient meal service normally begins at 7:30 A.M., so Donna and her staff have 90 minutes to develop a plan for breakfast. All of the stovetops, ovens, serving steam tables, and toasters, as well as the coffeemaker and microwave, are dependent on electricity and are unavailable for use. The hospital does have a generator, but it is reserved for emergency lighting throughout the hospital and for healthcare equipment and machinery in the patient care areas.

The patient menu for the day was originally as follows:

Breakfast

Orange Juice
Scrambled Egg
Pancakes with Syrup
Toast   Bacon
Milk or Coffee

Lunch

Tomato Soup with Saltines
Grilled Ham and Cheese Sandwich
Steamed Carrots
Fresh Fruit Cup
Oatmeal Cookies
Lemonade or Milk

Dinner

Coleslaw   Corn Chowder
BBQ Chicken
French Fries
Green Beans with Almonds
Chocolate Cake
Dinner Roll   Iced Tea

Donna's task is to plan menus based on the minimum levels suggested by the Food Guide Pyramid guidelines. She would also like to provide foods similar to the ones that were on the original menu, to best meet the customers' preferences.

Meals for the day will need to provide *at least:*

6 servings of bread, rice, pasta, cereal, grains

2 servings of fruits

3 servings of vegetables

2 servings of milk/dairy

2 servings of meat or protein

fats and sweets, sparingly

Donna and her staff are able to use items in the refrigerator, such as milk, cheese, lunchmeat, and produce. Items in the freezer are useless, except ice cream (remember there are no methods to heat any foods). All other food choices will need to be nonperishable (canned, jarred, dried, bagged, boxed) and items with a short shelf life, such as breads, pastries, cakes, cookies. The staff does have access to clean running water. Unfortunately, the dishwasher runs on electric current.

Questions

1. For each menu item, determine whether it still can be served based on the information above. If it cannot, list another item that could be served and would be appropriate. (Hint: Substitute another type of appetizer, such as a mixed olive and mushroom salad instead of fried mushrooms. Or serve a tuna salad sandwich instead of a fried fish sandwich.)

   Orange juice: _____   Scrambled egg: _____
   Pancake/syrup: _____   Toast: _____
   Bacon: _____   Milk: _____
   Coffee: _____

   Tomato soup/saltines: _____ Grilled ham and cheese: _____
   Steamed carrots: _____   Fresh fruit cup: _____
   Oatmeal cookies: _____   Lemonade: _____
   Milk: _____

   Coleslaw: _____   Corn chowder: _____
   BBQ chicken: _____   French fries: _____
   Green beans/almonds: _____   Chocolate cake: _____
   Dinner roll: _____   Iced tea: _____

2. Based on your suggestions above, make sure you meet the Food Guide Pyramid recommendations. Categorize menu choices below:

   6 breads/rices/pastas/cereals/grains _____
   2 fruits _____
   3 vegetables _____
   2 milk or dairy _____
   2 meats or proteins _____
   fats and sweets _____

3. It is time to assemble the patient meal trays. With your dishwasher not working, what changes might you make in service? How will cleanup after the meal differ when the patient trays are returned to the dish room?

4. Obviously, the patients in the hospital will know the power is out. What might you want them to know about the change in meal service? How will you communicate this to each patient?

5. Based on this exercise, list *nonperishable* items that the manager could keep on the shelf at all times in case of an extended emergency. (You would not be able to use refrigerated items after about one day without power.) Keep in mind the Food Guide Pyramid, as well as the need to choose items that can be used on a daily basis and do not occupy shelf space for a rare emergency. List at least five items for each category. Remember, no heating!

Bread/rice/pasta/cereal/grains: _____
Fruits: _____
Vegetables: _____
Milk or dairy: _____
Meat or protein: _____
Fats and sweets: _____

Reference

U.S. Department of Agriculture. October 1996. The food guide pyramid. *Home and Garden Bulletin.* no. 252: Revised. August 1992.

Cases in Purchasing

STRATEGIES FOR DEALING WITH FOOD SHORTAGES

METRO NORTH COLLABORATIVE: A SCHOOL FOOD SERVICE PURCHASING SOLUTION

PURCHASING WITH PAR LEVELS

PROVISION OF NONCHARGE FORMULA PREPARATION AND ORAL FEEDING SUPPLIES

Strategies for Dealing with Food Shortages

Objectives

At the completion of this case study, students should be able to:

1. Identify the short- and long-term problems associated with shortages of food items at delivery.
2. Recognize the need for record keeping if food wholesalers are to be held accountable for their actions.
3. Identify the considerations that need to be taken into account when making menu item substitutions.

Case Narrative

Jackie is the manager of a small nursing home food service facility in Chicago. The facility uses six major vendors as follows:

- Produce: Bartlett and Sons Produce Wholesalers
- Staple items: Somerset Food Wholesalers
- Dairy: Klemmer's Dairy Wholesalers
- Meats: Porter's Quality Meats
- Bakery: Brenner's Baked Goods

Other vendors are used as necessary to meet the needs of the facility. The facility uses a just-in-time inventory system since its storage space is very limited. Recently Jackie reviewed the results of a client survey that she had conducted a few days previously. On the survey, one of her clients indicated that he had ordered the fried chicken dinner with cauliflower the previous evening and was sent broccoli instead of the cauliflower. Jackie wondered why the facility would run out of cauliflower on that evening and called the head chef to inquire. The head chef, Larry, explained that Bartlett's Produce Wholesaler was out of the item and there wasn't time to order it from another company. He chose to substitute broccoli for the cauliflower, but this meant that there wasn't enough broccoli for the broccoli and tomato salad that is a favorite among both clients and staff. Jackie asked whether being shorted on items (items ordered but not delivered as requested) was a common problem with the produce company or any other wholesalers. Larry reported that he wasn't sure whether the shortage rate was unusually high, but that it does happen on occasion. He went on to say that he didn't think that there were as many shortages last year, when they were using Sutton Produce Wholesalers. Jackie then asked why the broccoli was used as a substitute, Larry responded that most individuals who like cauliflower also like broccoli, so it seemed to make sense at the time. He went on to explain that he didn't realize the cauliflower was missing from the order until the dinner meal production had begun so he couldn't order extra broccoli to cover both menu needs.

To prevent having to make substitutions in the future, Jackie recommended that Larry order the frozen version of the major vegetables and keep them on hand for just such a situation. Larry reluctantly agreed but pointed out that shortages are not always in the produce area. Just last week Somerset Wholesalers shorted them on cornmeal, and thus they had no cornbread for the menu for two days. Jackie considered talking to the wholesalers in general to stress the importance of filling orders without shortages or substitutions, but she wasn't sure exactly what she should say.

Questions

1. Was broccoli a good choice as a substitution for cauliflower on this menu? Why or why not?
2. How might the handling of this specific food item shortage be improved?
3. What are the pros and cons of ordering frozen vegetables as backup in case fresh items are not available?
4. What should Jackie say to the wholesalers, if anything, with regard to shortages?
5. What should Jackie do to determine whether the shortage rate really is unacceptable, and, if so, how could she reduce the shortage rate?

Metro North Collaborative

A School Food Service Purchasing Solution

Objectives

At the completion of this case study, students should be able to:

1. Describe a cooperative method of procurement.
2. Identify some of the challenges and benefits of a cooperative or collaborative purchasing program.

Case Narrative

Collaborative purchasing for school food service programs is the process by which two or more school food authorities (SFAs) join together to establish an organization that subsequently publishes a Request for Bid (RFB) to purchase food and/or nonfood supplies for member SFAs.

The Metro North Collaborative was formed when numerous food service directors from public school districts in an area north of Boston, Massachusetts, began to question their ability to purchase food and supplies in a cost-effective manner. Several of the directors had been members of The Educational Cooperative (TEC), which operated for the benefit of school districts just west of Boston. At one point, TEC bid responses for bread and dairy products rose to very high levels, and when vendors were questioned as to the dramatic increase in pricing, they cited the extensive delivery requirements by the geographically widespread members included in the bid.

Objectives of the Metro North Collaborative

The Metro North Collaborative developed the following objectives to meet the needs of its members:

- To bid collectively for products and services used by the food service departments of member school districts
- To ensure competitive and equitable pricing for all member districts
- To ensure bid compliance with the letter and spirit of Commonwealth of Massachusetts Public Procurement Laws under M.G.L. c. 30B, The Uniform Procurement Act
- To provide member food service directors with peer support in the operation of school nutrition programs
- To provide professional development, especially in the area of public procurement regulations as they relate to the purchase of food and supplies used by member food service departments
- To promote the importance of school nutrition programs in the development of healthy students nutritionally, socially, physically, and psychologically

Formal Establishment of the Metro North Collaborative

Due to problems of serving a wide geographic distribution with bread and dairy vendors, it was decided that members would be limited to a specific geographic area north of Boston. Invitational meetings were held, with all public school food service directors within the delineated geographic area contacted and invited to participate in the collaborative.

A public purchasing agent from one of the member towns, as well as a representative from the Massachusetts Department of Education, Nutrition Programs and Services, became advisors. Bids were written for dairy products and bread products, with documents added for a limited number of groceries in subsequent years. It took eight years of bidding experience before the group felt comfortable with the concept of a large grocery bid. Finally, in the year 2000, a formal organizational structure was adopted (Figure 1).

Rationale for Collaborative Bidding

In most states, public agencies *must* follow bidding regulations or laws that define a relationship between the purchasing institution and the vendor. In Massachusetts, these agencies, including all public schools, must comply with Chapter 30B of the Massachusetts Public Laws. The Massachusetts Office of the Inspector General oversees compliance with these bidding regulations. The bidding process can be very time consuming. Dividing the effort among collaborative members saves many hours of work for each food service director.

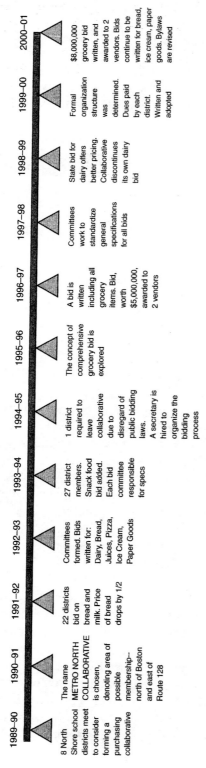

1989–90
8 North Shore school districts meet to consider forming a purchasing collaborative

1990–91
The name METRO NORTH COLLABORATIVE is chosen, denoting area of possible membership—north of Boston and east of Route 128

1991–92
22 districts bid on bread and milk. Price of bread drops by 1/2

1992–93
Committees formed. Bids written for: Dairy, Bread, Juices, Pizza, Ice Cream, Paper Goods

1993–94
27 district members. Snack food bid added. Each bid committee responsible for specs

1994–95
1 district required to leave collaborative due to disregard of public bidding laws. A secretary is hired to organize the bidding process

1995–96
The concept of comprehensive grocery bid is explored

1996–97
A bid is written including all grocery items. Bid, worth $5,000,000, awarded to 2 vendors

1997–98
Committees work to standardize general specifications for all bids

1998–99
State bid for dairy offers better pricing. Collaborative discontinues its own dairy bid

1999–00
Formal organization structure was determined. Dues paid by each district. Written and adopted

2000–01
$8,000,000 grocery bid written, and awarded to 2 vendors. Bids continue to be written for bread, ice cream, paper goods. Bylaws are revised

Figure 2–1   Evolution of Metro North Collaborative

25

One of the main purposes of cooperative purchasing is to enable school districts to save money. By joining together, school districts can increase their buying power. Ten school districts with four schools each can have the same buying leverage as a forty-school district. Smaller, independent institutions do not have the large product usage numbers to command the most favorable pricing structures from vendors and manufacturers.

An added benefit of collaborative purchasing is the information exchange within the area. It tends to increase standardization of procedures and specifications. The more uniform these features are, the easier it is for vendors to deal with schools. This increases the collaborative's desirability as a customer, and vendors frequently work harder to keep their business.

Keys to Successful Collaborative Bidding

Successful collaborative bidding includes the following key points:

- Know local bidding regulations. Local regulations may differ from state codes in relation to several aspects of financial limits. Local regulations take precedence over state codes.
- Research local and statewide bids that may be available and may provide advantageous pricing and specifications.
- Ask for advice from experienced purchasing professionals. The institution or political subdivision may employ purchasing professionals.
- Research which agency controls or advises institutions on the bidding process in a state.
- Begin the bidding process on a limited number of easily specified items. Milk is the easiest food product to begin with. It has a limited number of standard specifications that are clearly definable and agreed upon by users and vendors alike.
- Define product specifications clearly, by testing numerous available products and agreeing to use as few variations as possible.
- Be realistic in specifications. (For example, do not demand a $100 minimum grocery delivery when all vendors in the area already require a much higher threshold. It will discourage viable vendors from responding to a bid.)
- Collaborate with similar types of institutions. Although the same principals can be adapted to any type of public food service operation, it is less complicated if comparable institutions collaborate since they generally use similar products. (For example, public schools, residential schools, public hospitals, or public long-term care institutions, each should collaborate separately with like institutions.)
- Set definitive parameters for maintaining active membership.

- Determine whether paid staff will be employed or collaborative members will divide up the administrative and clerical tasks.
- Define an organizational plan and bylaws.
- Hold all members to the same standards, especially when dealing with vendors and observing regulations.
- Reevaluate bids, specifications, and policies on a regular basis.

Areas Where Problems May Arise

Product Specifications. It is very difficult for all members to agree on specifications for each product. Each district has "favorite" products or foods that are more popular there than in another district. To reach agreement on specifications, hold a taste testing and can cuttings using specific, measurable criteria. A good specification includes the following elements:

- a short, clearly written description of the desired product
- the quality of the product, using either U.S. Department of Agriculture or industry standards
- the pack size desired, expressed in can size, pounds, etc.
- if known, the desired yield per unit, expressed in terms of can count and drained weight
- characteristics that are generally standard and recognizable within the food industry.

A good specification does not necessarily state manufacturer and product code, unless that is the *only* way to adequately describe the desired product. A vendor may:

- not bid if the specified brand is not available, even though an equivalent or superior product may be available at an equal or better price
- have a favorable relationship with a manufacturer who is unknown to the collaborative. By specifying a brand name, a superior product or vendor may be eliminated unintentionally.

If a collaborative can guarantee a vendor a large quantity of a particular food from one manufacturer, the vendor can often secure a lower price from the manufacturer.

Open-ended specifications can cause confusion among collaborative members and potential bid respondents. For example, most vendors have minimum delivery requirements. They may be stated in dollar amounts or case quantities, and they require either a service charge or refusal of delivery if minimum amounts are not met. If the minimums are stated *by the collaborative* as a specification in the bid document, any vendor altering the bid by stating a different amount cannot be considered a "responsive" vendor.

Vendor Relationships. Some members may have long-term relationships with vendors and may expect "special" treatment, which, in a public bidding relationship, is generally *not* legal. Specify in the bid any allowance or special consideration offered to high-volume users. These may include volume discounts per delivery or percentage reduction in total purchases, but they should not be the basis for bid award.

Work Load. A few members tend to shoulder much of the work burden. A provision for committee service for each member should be specified in the bylaws or operational contract.

Bid Award. A single award to one prime grocery vendor can cause that distributor to become complacent. Consider multiple or dual awards allowing members to purchase from any or all approved vendors. This encourages price and service competition among vendors.

Conclusion

There are both advantages and disadvantages to the formation of a collaborative food service purchasing group. Although there are differences of opinion in every newly created group, to be successful the group must be cohesive and cooperative. All members must work together toward a common set of goals. The principal benefits of collaborative purchasing are the savings of time in the bid preparation process and the advantageous pricing that occurs when small, independent institutions purchase as a unit.

Questions

It took an entire year for a school food service collaborative to develop a grocery bid. More than 300 items were specified and bid. The bid was awarded to two grocery vendors. One of the vendors was regional in scope, the other was a division of a very large national distributor.

The food service director from one of the member districts discovered, *after the bid was awarded and contracts were signed,* that the chicken nuggets that were available for purchase through the bid were completely different from the ones with which her students were familiar. She was concerned that students would not participate in the lunch program if she changed the product.

1. What can the food service director do *under the existing bid* to provide product that her students will eat?
2. Describe the steps the food service director could have taken *during the bid-writing process* to assure that the products available for purchase met the needs of the department?

Internet References for Use in the Process of Public Bidding

http://www.foodprofile.com/main/index.htm
http://profileshowcase.foodprofile.com/internetshowcase/default_sman.htm
http://www.mass.gov/agency/documents/osd/policy/phand.pdf
http://admin.state.nh.us/purchasing/
http://www.nfsmi.org/Education/Satellite/ss16/parthand.pdf

Purchasing with Par Levels

Objectives

At the completion of this case study, students should be able to:

1. Identify what a par level is in regard to food inventory and purchasing.
2. Use quantity recipes, along with par levels, to prepare a sample order for purchasing goods.
3. Identify typical food items that are kept at par levels because of their frequent usage.

Case Narrative

Greg is performing the weekly food and supply order at Glen Maple Hospital. The hospital serves patient meals and has a cafeteria for staff and visitors. Greg receives one delivery each week from his primary vendor and two produce deliveries each week. The inventory and food usage system used at Glen Maple is called the FIFO (First In, First Out) system. Goods that are received each week are physically stored behind food products currently on the shelf, so the oldest goods are used first. This method ensures fresher quality and less waste due to old product spoilage. The FIFO system is most important with perishable food items.

Greg keeps par levels for goods that are used frequently. A par level is the lowest amount of a food product that should be on the shelf at any given time. It is a "safety net" so that Greg will not run out of a food product that is used often. Examples of foods that commonly have par levels are: coffee, flour, eggs, milk, juices, and meats that are used frequently, such as hamburger or chicken. Greg's hospital serves several hundred orders of french fries in the cafeteria each week, so he has a par level of three cases of fries in his freezer. A salad bar is offered daily in the cafeteria, and Greg uses about four cases of lettuce per week so he has a par level of one case of lettuce. In addition to the par levels, Greg must order what he predicts he will need for the menu items that will be prepared by the chef that week. This week Chef Jim is preparing spaghetti with meat sauce on Wednesday, a popular menu item. The ingredients needed for the meat sauce recipe, which serves 200, are as follows:

7 No. 10 cans of tomato puree
1 No. 10 can of tomato paste
50 lb. ground beef
5 cans canned mushrooms (No. 303)
4 lb. white or yellow onions, chopped
½ c. dried basil
4 Tablespoon salt

Chef Jim is also preparing Chicken Italiano (100 servings):

3 No. 10 cans of tomato puree
32 oz. Italian salad dressing
6 lb. shredded mozzarella cheese
100 6 oz. chicken breasts, boneless/skinless

Greg keeps par levels on the following products used in the two recipes:

Tomato puree, No. 10	6 cans (1 case)
Tomato paste, No. 10	3 cans (½ case)
Ground beef, 1 lb. slabs	40 lb. (1 case)
Canned mushrooms, No. 303	12 cans (⅓ case)
Onions, 50 lb. sack	25 lb. (½ sack)
Italian dressing, gallon	1 gallon (¼ case)
Mozzarella cheese, 2 lb. bag	2 bags (½ case)
Chicken breasts, boneless/skinless, 6 oz.	24 pieces (1 case)

As Greg performs his inventory, he notes the following products on the shelf, in the refrigerator, and in the freezer:

Tomato puree, No. 10	4 cans
Tomato paste, No. 10	2 cans

Ground beef, 40 lb. case	60 lb. (1½ cases)
Canned mushrooms, No. 303	22 cans
Onions, 50 lb. sack	12½ lb. (¼ sack)
Italian dressing, gallon	3 gallons
Mozzarella cheese, 2 lb. bag	2 bags
Chicken breasts, boneless/skinless, 6 oz.	10 pieces (¾ case)

Questions

1. Based on Greg's par levels and the needs for both recipes, fill in the order.

   Par + Qty needed for recipe − inventory = Qty to order
   Qty to order ÷ Number per case = Cases to order (round to whole number)

   Be sure to *order by the case.*

Item / number per case	Par / Qty needed	Inventory (on hand)	Qty to order	Cases to order
Tomato puree / 6	6+	4		
Tomato paste / 6	3+	2		
Mushrooms / 36	12+	22		
Italian dressing / 4	1+	3		
Onion / 50 lb. sack	25 lb.+	¼ sack		
Mozzarella / 4	2+	2		
Ground beef / 40 lb.	40 lb.+	60 lb.		
Chicken, 6 oz. / 24 ea.	24+	10		

2. Par levels are established for foods that are used in large volume. Name four foods that would have high par levels in each of the following establishments:

   Fast food: _____
   Mexican dining: _____
   Chinese dining: _____
   Pancake house: _____

3. As Greg did inventory, he noticed his storeroom employee had put new tomato puree in front of cans that were older and already on the shelf. What organizational methods can be implemented so that the FIFO system is followed?

4. Name at least three items for which you *would not* establish par levels.

Provision of Noncharge Formula Preparation and Oral Feeding Supplies

Objectives

At the completion of this case study, students should be able to:

1. Choose a replacement product for a major supply item, ensuring uninterrupted service at best cost.
2. Plan negotiations with vendors to ensure product availability and maintain good relations.

Case Narrative

In Montgomery Pediatrics Hospital, a pediatric acute-care facility, about one-third of the patients require some sort of formula: either canned enteral products, ready-to-feed infant nursettes, or formulas reconstituted from powder. Almost 70 percent of the formula needs are met by canned enterals and infant nursettes. The remainder of the formula is prepared from powder in a centralized formula preparation room and delivered to the appropriate unit. Many patients who are receiving formula also use oral feeding supplies such as bottles and nipples.

In the formula preparation process, sterilized water is used to reconstitute powdered formula. (Enough formula is made for a twenty-four-hour supply for the patient.) Once prepared, formula is poured into the glass bottles that the sterilized water was packaged in. These bottles are relabeled and delivered to the floors. Some sterilized water is also stocked in the units for use in diluting breast milk and enteral formula.

The sterilized water is packaged in four-ounce glass bottles and is currently provided at no charge by a formula manufacturer (Company A). Another formula manufacturer (Company B) produces sterilized water in three-ounce glass bottles, which they are also willing to provide at no cost. Furthermore, both of these companies provide other feeding supplies at no charge, as included in Table 1. Both companies manufacture essentially the same formula preparation and feeding supplies. The majority of the supplies are provided by Company A because, up until the last few years, the facility contracted to purchase 80 percent of the formula from them. In the last few years the facility expanded its formulary and thus did not renew the contract with Company A, but it did continue to receive most of the noncharge items from them.

In an attempt to control costs, Company A recently announced a few changes:

- They will be manufacturing sterilized water in two-ounce plastic bottles rather than four-ounce glass bottles.
- They are cutting the number of bottles of sterilized water that they will provide in half. Since the bottles will be half the size, the facility will actually receive one-fourth as much water as they do currently.
- They are also reducing the amount of the other noncharge feeding supplies they provide to meet approximately half of the facility's needs.

The two-ounce bottles of sterilized water are tall and narrow, and it is difficult to pour into them. In addition, they do not fit as well on the shelves or in the

Table 1   Feeding Supplies

Company	Product	Amount used/year[*]	Cost to company[*]
A			
	Sterilized water	48,000 bottles for formula prep	$0.75 per bottle
		9,600 bottles stocked on units	$0.75 per bottle
	Disposable plastic bottles		
	2 ounce	73,000 bottles	$0.50 per bottle
	8 ounce	18,720 bottles	$1.00 per bottle
	Disposable nipples		
	Regular	91,250 nipples	$0.15 per nipple
	Orthodontic	13,000 nipples	$0.25 per nipple
	Premature	26,000 nipples	$0.25 per nipple
B			
	Disposable nipples		
	Regular	3,000 nipples	$0.15 per nipple
	Orthodontic	13,000 nipples	$0.25 per nipple

[*]Not actual amounts or costs—proprietary information.

refrigerators; however, the company has offered to offset the costs of moving shelves and buying new containers to accommodate the new bottle size. Even though they are half the size, the cost of the two-ounce bottles of sterilized water is the same per bottle as the cost of the four-ounce bottles.

Company B will provide formula preparation and feeding supplies at no charge to meet up to half of the facility's needs. The three-ounce bottles of sterilized water they provide are almost as easy to pour into as the four-ounce bottles, are a similar shape, and are approximately the same cost per bottle. Their other oral feeding supplies are nearly identical to those provided by Company A.

Questions

1. What are some options to replace the four-ounce bottle of sterilized water for formula preparation? What is the best choice?
2. What possible solutions might be negotiated with each company concerning formula preparation and oral feeding supplies?
3. In what areas might costs increase, and what could be done to adjust for that?
4. What must be done to maintain good relations with the formula companies and to ensure product availability?

Cases in Food Production

Dealing with Your Boss's Unrealistic Expectations

Objectives

At the completion of this case study, students should be able to:

1. Identify some of the many factors influencing patient acceptance of food.
2. Strategize about means for clarifying patient food acceptance issues.
3. Debate the merits of catering to the wealthy client.

Case Narrative

Sharika is the chief dietitian at St. Catherine's Community Hospital. She was working on the employee schedule in her office one day when the head administrator, Bob Jackson, came by to speak to her. He told Sharika that Mrs. Valencia Wellstone, a very wealthy woman and possible benefactor, had just been admitted to the sixth floor. He strongly expressed the need for special treatment and told Sharika that she should provide Mrs. Wellstone with any food she desired and should deliver all of Mrs. Wellstone's meals personally. Sharika was taken aback by this expectation and asked what should be done on her days off. Bob informed Sharika that there would be no days off while Mrs. Wellstone was in the hospital. He indicated that Mrs. Wellstone had the potential to donate a large sum of money to the hospital and her stay at the facility must be as favorable as possible. Sharika asked what the admitting diagnosis and diet order was, and Bob did not know.

After Bob left, Sharika sighed. She had so much work to do already, and there were plenty of low-income patients in the hospital who really needed intervention since they would not be able to afford healthcare once they were discharged. She shrugged and made her way up to the sixth floor to talk to Mrs. Wellstone.

When she checked the chart, she saw that Mrs. Wellstone was admitted for difficulty in breathing secondary to metastatic lung cancer. She had been prescribed myriad drugs and was receiving chemotherapy. Luckily, she was placed on a regular diet. Admission notes indicated that Mrs. Wellstone lived in New York but was visiting Miami when her acute symptoms occurred. A knot formed in Sharika's stomach because she knew this patient had a poor prognosis and was not likely to feel much like eating. She went in to talk to Mrs. Wellstone and found that she was accompanied by her full-time caregiver and aide, Maria Gomez. Sharika asked Mrs. Wellstone how she was feeling. Mrs. Wellstone replied that she was tired and disappointed to be in a hospital so far from home. Sharika obtained food preferences from Mrs. Wellstone and developed some menus based on those preferences, which Mrs. Wellstone approved.

Over the course of the next seven days, Sharika brought all the food trays to Mrs. Wellstone and had special meals prepared to her liking, some of which required the purchase of special foods from local markets. The chefs were actually enjoying the chance to make some more difficult and interesting food items, but it certainly put a strain on staffing. Sharika enjoyed getting to know Mrs. Wellstone but felt frustrated by the need to deliver all the trays. She would often have to leave a diet instruction or consultation before it was completed so she could pick up the food tray for Mrs. Wellstone from the kitchen and deliver it to her. On two occasions, she forgot temporarily and the tray was sitting in the kitchen longer than desired.

On day seven, Bob stopped in to see Sharika. He explained that Mrs. Wellstone was complaining about the food to her assistant and a nurse overheard the conversation. Bob seemed visibly upset and was using an accusatory tone of voice. He stated in no uncertain terms that Sharika needed to rectify this situation and finished his diatribe with, "If you can't provide food that is acceptable to Mrs. Wellstone, I'm sure we can find someone else who will!"

Sharika was stunned. She immediately went up to talk to Maria Gomez, Mrs. Wellstone's caregiver. Maria stated that Mrs. Wellstone was very depressed and her health was failing. Sharika had checked the medical record prior to the visit and it confirmed the downward trend. When Sharika asked about Mrs. Wellstone's satisfaction with the food, Maria indicated that there wasn't much that could make Mrs. Wellstone happy right now. She admitted that her food consumption had dropped and she was really just nibbling at her meals. Sharika took Mrs. Wellstone's hand and asked her if there was anything more she could do for her. Mrs. Wellstone simply said she was fine and needed to rest.

Sharika returned to her office, totally frustrated. She couldn't imagine what she could do to improve Mrs. Wellstone's perception of the food and felt her job was at stake. What in the world should she do?

Questions

1. Is Mrs. Wellstone's lack of satisfaction with the food a good indicator of the food quality? What else might be influencing her perceptions of the food?
2. Was it a good decision to have Sharika deliver the trays to Mrs. Wellstone rather than having the regular hosts and hostesses deliver them? Defend your answer.
3. How can Sharika make sure she does not forget to deliver the trays to Mrs. Wellstone as soon as they are ready?
4. What specific problems does Sharika face at this point?
5. What should she do to address this difficult situation?
6. How might employees react to the obvious "special treatment" this wealthy patient is receiving? Can this practice be defended?

Managing Food Service Production and Forecasting

Fried Chicken Friday at Glen Maple Hospital

Objectives

At the completion of this case study, students should be able to:

1. Calculate production needs for a multi-unit operation based on historical forecasting.
2. Problem solve solutions to overages or shortages in the food service operation.

Case Narrative

It is 12:30 Friday afternoon. Chef Jim is checking quantities of fried chicken on the patient tray line and the cafeteria serving line. The patient tray line will run for approximately thirty more minutes, during which time seventy-five more trays will be prepared. The cafeteria hours of service are from 11:00 A.M. to 1:30 P.M.

Based on Jim's forecasting sheets, he knows the following history on popular "Fried Chicken Friday":

- Approximately 65 percent of cafeteria customers purchase the chicken on Friday.
- The average number of customers on Friday is 470.
- Approximately 45 percent of patients order the fried chicken from their menu.

Today, there are 280 patients in the hospital. Of those 280 patients:

- 210 are eating solid foods
- 18 patients are on liquid only diets
- 52 patients are NPO, and receive nothing to eat

42

Out of the 210 patients eating solid foods, 125 are on specialty diets: heart healthy, low fat, low salt, or diabetic. They are not offered the fried chicken on their menu.

Chef Jim notes that there are fifteen pieces of fried chicken in the cafeteria on the service line. Chef Jim just prepared another thirty pieces, which are being held in a warmer. There is still 1 case (sixty pieces) of raw chicken in the prep area. There are ten pieces of fried chicken on the patient tray line at 12:30 P.M.

Questions

Show all of your calculations.

1. a. How many pieces of chicken did Chef Jim need to prepare for the cafeteria customers for the entire lunch service, based on his forecasting sheets and history?
   b. How many pieces of chicken did Jim need to prepare to meet the patient tray line needs for the entire lunch service, based on his history and forecasting?
2. After 12:30 P.M., approximately how many pieces of chicken will be sold in the cafeteria before closing time? (Assume that the flow of customers is steady from 11:00 A.M. to 1:30 P.M.)
3. At 12:30 P.M., approximately how many pieces of chicken will be needed to complete the patient tray line, based on forecasting?
4. How many pieces of chicken are potentially available (both cooked and raw) at 12:30 P.M. to cover the needs of both the cafeteria and the patient tray line? Will Chef Jim be over or under on his forecast, and by how many pieces?
5. Based on your findings, what would *you* do if you were Chef Jim? What might you do in the future when the same menu is featured?
6. a. What is the financial impact of overproduction for Chef Jim?
   b. What is the impact to customer satisfaction if there is underproduction?

Forecasting Surprise

Objectives

At the completion of the case study, students should be able to:

1. List routine information sources used to forecast production needs.
2. Evaluate alternative information sources.
3. Adjust forecasted production volumes based on all information received.

Case Narrative

This case study takes place in a medium-sized hospital in an urban area. The food service department runs a fairly popular cafeteria service seven days a week. Many hospital staff members, physicians, office personnel from the nearby doctors' office complex, visitors, and family members of the patients buy meals or snack items throughout the day. The hospital cafeteria has developed a community reputation over the years as a good place to have a nice meal at a reasonable price. The cafeteria competes with several nice restaurants within walking distance from the hospital; however, the prices are significantly higher at these restaurants and the cafeteria is a much quicker option for shift workers with only a thirty-minute meal break.

To maintain quality and keep his prices reasonable, the manager and his cooking staff work diligently to hold excess production to a minimum. Their community reputation would be jeopardized if they ran out of an item during a meal. To make the most accurate production forecast possible, the kitchen manager regularly reviews cafeteria sales records for each of the cafeteria menus used, the local newspapers for current events, and current weather reports. He also evaluates the

44

popularity of specific items when those items compete with each other at the same meal by reviewing the past sales records when those items were both on the same day's menu.

Tomorrow's cafeteria menu offers southern fried chicken, sliced roast beef with gravy, and a tuna salad cold plate as entrées. In the previous menu cycle, 53 percent of the cafeteria patrons had selected the southern fried chicken, 32 percent had selected the sliced roast beef with gravy, and about 15 percent had selected the tuna salad cold plate. The manager noted that the weather conditions were similar to the previous menu cycle and there were no special events or holidays occurring during this cycle. The manager and the cooks decided to forecast the food production at 55 percent of the total number of sales for southern fried chicken, 34 percent for the sliced roast beef with gravy, and 16 percent for the tuna salad cold plate. This would give the kitchen a 5 percent padded production volume.

On the day of the southern fried chicken, sliced roast beef with gravy, and a tuna salad cold plate lunch the manager received some surprising news. As the manager got his morning coffee, the cafeteria cashier told him that a number of office nurses who had been in the cafeteria earlier were talking about a weight-loss diet emphasizing fish. The cashier commented that the office nurses were delighted that tuna was on the menu for today.

As the manager walked back through the kitchen to his office, he overheard several of his aides returning from taking the breakfast carts to the nursing units telling the cooks about this "hot new low-cal diet" that is starting today all over the building. One aide said excitedly, "Like it was like everywhere, Dude! Everybody is starting this new low-calorie diet today that makes you like eat fish like all the time!"

Questions

1. Would the cafeteria cashier and the dietary aides be reliable sources of forecasting information? Explain why or why not.
2. Should the manager and cooks reevaluate the production amounts of southern fried chicken, sliced roast beef with gravy, and a tuna salad cold plate? Explain why or why not.
3. Given this new information and using the padded percentages forecasted for the southern fried chicken, sliced roast beef with gravy, and tuna salad cold plate, forecast the potential cafeteria lunch production needs.
4. Would you make any changes in the menus for upcoming days based on this information?
5. How might forecasting for this meal be affected by a weather forecast of winds and heavy rain?
6. How might the forecasted amounts for this meal change if it were payday and paychecks were largely direct deposit?

Cases in Service

Evaluation of Patient Satisfaction Using Two Different Tray Systems

Objectives

At the completion of this case study, students should be able to:

1. Identify factors that may hinder optimal performance of food delivery systems.
2. Identify factors that may influence an institution's decision to choose a standard versus a covered tray.

Case Narrative

A Department of Veterans Affairs Medical Center (DVAMC) in the Midwest is a two-division medical center with 232 hospital beds, 71 nursing home care unit beds, and 50 domiciliary beds. The Lee Adams (LA) Division is the center for acute medical and surgical care and has 132 operating hospital beds. The Marcus Mahoney (MM) Division is the center for the nursing home unit and the domiciliary. The MM Division also has 100 inpatient beds that provide services to patients in acute psychiatric care, spinal cord injury, and rehabilitative services. In addition, MM is the primary site of food production.

The food production system at this Veterans Affairs (VA) facility is a traditional cook and serve system. A three-week-cycle, nonselective menu is used. All of the food is produced in one centralized kitchen at MM, and then transported to three decentralized kitchens, one servicing LA and two servicing MM. The decentralized kitchen at LA services all of the inpatients in one building, while the two decentralized kitchens at MM service three inpatient buildings.

Patient satisfaction surveys in the spinal cord injury unit have consistently revealed low patient satisfaction, especially in the area of food temperature. Factors that are likely to affect overall patient satisfaction in the spinal cord injury unit include increased length of hospital stay and a high frequency of rehospitalization. However, low satisfaction for food temperature was of particular concern for the food service manager. Proper food temperature is critical for patient safety. [Some research has also shown that taste of food as well as food temperatures have a great impact on overall patient satisfaction.]

Part One

A factor contributing to decreased patient satisfaction in the area of food temperature may be the increased transportation time to the spinal cord injury unit. Because the spinal cord injury unit is the only inpatient unit without its own kitchen, food is transported from a decentralized kitchen in another building. Currently, the standard "heat on demand" system is employed throughout the DVAMC. The food service manager was interested in learning whether the covered tray system might improve food temperature and therefore improve patient satisfaction. Because patient satisfaction scores were much higher among other inpatient areas of the hospital, the food service manager was considering using the covered tray system only for the spinal cord injury unit. If food temperature retention was significantly better, she also considered the possibility of converting the entire standard tray system to a covered tray system. This might allow her to consolidate to one decentralized kitchen at MM and would eventually save money on labor and equipment.

Question

How might you set up a study assessing food temperatures and other attributes of these two systems?

Part Two

A covered tray system was loaned out to the DVAMC so a temperature study could be done. In order to evaluate the effectiveness of the standard tray versus the covered tray system, both types of trays were used during one meal and temperatures were taken as follows:

- food in the steam table at the start, middle, and completion of service
- plates as they were removed from the plate lowerator (warmer)
- plated food as it left the tray line
- plated food as it arrived on the patient unit

The elapsed time between when the food left the tray line and when the food was finally served was also recorded. Patient satisfaction responses from each of the systems were compared.

Problems with food temperatures were identified immediately. On four different trials, plate temperature measurements ranged from 87 to 94 degrees Fahrenheit. This temperature range fell far below the required 150 to 175 degrees Fahrenheit needed for optimal performance of the standard heat on demand system. Furthermore, although food was at an appropriate temperature in the steam tables, it was found that once food was plated, the temperatures did not meet VA standards. Once plate temperatures were corrected, there were no significant differences between the final food temperatures of the standard versus the covered tray systems.

Patient satisfaction surveys in the spinal cord injury unit revealed that the patients who received their meals on the covered tray system gave higher satisfaction scores for food temperature. They also thought the food looked more appealing on the compartmentalized tray, and they reported that the food tasted good. However, some problems with the covered tray system did exist. Many patients on the spinal cord injury unit received additional oral supplements to meet nutritional needs. There was not enough room for these supplements on the covered tray. In some instances, there also was some difficulty with the lid fitting securely on the plate due to the height of the food.

Questions

1. What considerations are required before choosing a tray system in a hospital-based food service system?
2. What effect, if any, did plate temperatures have on final food temperatures at time of service?
3. Why do you think patients gave higher satisfaction scores for foods they received on a covered tray than for foods they received on a standard tray?
4. Should the DVAMC switch to a covered tray system? Explain.

Internet Reference

www.aladdintemprite.com

References

Braverman S. P. *Review of dietetics, manual for the registered dietitian exam, 2003–2005.* Chicago: Hess & Hunt Inc.

O'Hara, P., D. Harper, M. Kangas, J. Dubeau, C. Borsutzky, and N. Lemire. 1997. Taste, temperature, and presentation predict satisfaction with foodservices in a Canadian continuing-care hospital. *Journal of the American Dietetic Association* 97, 401–406.

Rogers, M. 1996. Induction heats up patient meals. *Restaurants and Institutions* 106, 100.

Patient Complaint

Whose Hair Is This?

Objectives

At the completion of this case study, students should be able to:

1. Evaluate routine dietary employee hygiene policies and practices.
2. Evaluate standing policies and procedures regarding patient complaints and their investigations.
3. Evaluate the working relationships between other departments and the dietary staff.

Case Narrative

This patient complaint incident took place in a small hospital in a medium-sized town. The dietary department had a registered dietitian as its director and a retired military sergeant as the kitchen manager. The retired military sergeant had been trained in kitchen management by the military and ran the kitchen "by the book." The majority of the kitchen staff had worked for the hospital for many years and were well trained in the dress code, which included the use of hairnets.

On this particular day, all of the breakfast trays had been delivered to the patient care areas upstairs, and the cafeteria was doing a good business as usual for a weekday morning. The fully staffed kitchen was cleaning up from breakfast and starting lunch preparation when a phone call relaying a patient complaint and requesting a new breakfast tray was received from a nursing unit. The patient in room 206 had found hair in his breakfast eggs. A fresh tray was prepared, and both the dietary director and manager delivered the new tray to the patient in 206 after checking with the patient's nurse to confirm that he could still have a tray.

53

Upon entering the patient's room, the dietary director and manager introduced themselves and asked the patient to tell them what happened. The patient informed them that he was very angry when he found blonde hairs in his eggs. He threatened to sue the hospital. He demanded that this hospitalization be provided free to him because of this terrible incident. The dietary director and manager asked if they could have the first breakfast tray, which had the hairs in the eggs, so that they could investigate his concern more thoroughly. The patient reluctantly allowed them to have the breakfast tray that contained the hair. The dietary director and manager thanked the patient for his cooperation and assured him that they would look into this concern.

[*Before reading further in this case study, ask yourself what you would do next in this situation.*]

After the dietary director and manager left the patient's room, they asked to speak with the nurse currently in charge of the nursing unit involved in this patient complaint. They asked the charge nurse to furnish them with a list of all nursing employees currently working on the unit. As part of the information on the list, the charge nurse was to indicate which nursing staff passed breakfast trays and each person's hair color, as well as whether the hair was curly, straight, long, or short.

The dietary director and manager returned to the dietary department. The manager made a copy of the dietary employee schedule for the current week. He also made a list of each employee's name, hair color, and description of hair type (curly, straight, long, or short) and whether the employee was using a hair net. While the manager was compiling this information, the dietary director contacted the housekeeping director. A similar list of names and hair information was requested from the housekeeping staff that was working on the nursing unit that morning prior to or during the passing of the breakfast trays. The maintenance, laboratory, and radiology departments were also contacted for similar information.

Questions

1. Why did the dietary director and manager ask the patient to tell his own story?
2. Why was it important for the dietary director and manager to obtain the eggs with blonde hair?
3. Why did the dietary director and manager agree only to look into the patient's concern instead of accepting blame and apologizing for the incident?
4. Why did the dietary director and manager request information from the nursing, housekeeping, maintenance, laboratory, and radiology departments?

Customer Abuse of the "Cost per Serving Container" System

Objectives

At the completion of this case, students should be able to:

1. Describe one method of pricing food in a cafeteria.
2. Identify strengths and weaknesses of charging for items by the serving container size.
3. Recognize the ability of customers to use a given system to their own advantage.
4. Think critically about strategies for dealing with challenging customers.

Case Narrative

Martha was the food service director in a small hospital (forty beds, averaging 60 percent occupancy in a town of approximately eight thousand residents). Her operation included patient services, a cafeteria for employees and visitors, and several vending machines. The cafeteria had a small cafeteria line with two entrée, starch, and vegetable choices daily. A small salad bar also was provided in the dining room. Employees and customers were given a choice of dishes to "purchase" for the salad bar. The customer was charged $.35 for the small "monkey dish" bowl or $1.50 for a dinner plate. Clients paid for the plate and then helped themselves to the salad bar.

A year or so after starting the salad bar, Martha received a number of complaints about a particular employee. The complaint was that he was paying $.35 for the small monkey bowl, but making a meal out of it. Martha observed him on two occasions. He was an edgy, resourceful X-ray technician named Jack. He would take the small bowl and put potato salad in the center. Then he would prop celery and carrot sticks in the potato salad, around the edges, as a foundation. With those

55

in place, he proceeded to add a lot of salad, dressing, and other items available on the salad bar. By the time he was done, he had created a "masterpiece tower of food," up to ten inches high and three inches across!

After he had built this large salad in the small monkey dish, he would take a paper plate from the area next to the microwave (for employees that wanted to heat their own lunches), place it under his salad bowl, and dig in. With his first forkful, the salad piled high in the small bowl would tumble down and fill the plate. Thus, a full plateful of salad for $.35! No wonder other employees complained.

Questions

1. As food service director, how might you handle this situation?
2. What are some methods for preventing a similar incident with another employee in the future?
3. What are some other costing systems you could use? Identify the advantages and disadvantages of each of these systems.

Using the Performance Improvement Process to Address Late Tray Problems

Objectives

After completion of this case study, students should be able to:

1. Identify the benefit of engaging a multidisciplinary team to address a problem.
2. Use performance improvement tools, flow charts, and fishbone diagrams in describing work processes.
3. Describe the value of using the performance improvement process in food and nutrition services.

Case Narrative

The process for delivering food to patients in an acute hospital setting has not changed significantly over time. Most hospital food service operations assemble patient meals three times a day on an assembly or "tray" line and deliver meals to patients according to a delivery schedule established in collaboration with nursing. Patient care in acute care hospitals, however, has changed significantly in the past decade. Length of stay is much shorter and patient acuity is greater. Patients are away from their rooms for tests, procedures, and therapies causing them to miss their regularly scheduled meals. This case study describes one hospital's process to address this problem.

In an effort to establish a patient-centered care model, the hospital created a patient care technician (PCT) role. The concept was to have the same PCT interact with a few designated patients to perform a variety of tasks. One task included meal tray delivery. The Food and Nutrition Services department reduced their staff of tray passers to allow for an increase in full-time equivalents (FTEs) in nursing to establish the PCT role. One of the positions reduced was the individual responsible for delivering late trays to patients. Late trays are those meal or food items requested by patients in-between their regularly scheduled meal delivery periods.

The Food and Nutrition Services Department prepared the late trays, and it was the responsibility of the PCT to come and retrieve the tray from the kitchen and deliver it to the patient. There was a significant level of dissatisfaction expressed by the Nursing Department due to the amount of time the PCTs were away from the nursing unit. Monthly food and nutrition statistics indicated that there was an average of eight hundred late trays per month. The Food and Nutrition Services management also suspected that the number of late trays adversely affected patient satisfaction scores.

A performance improvement team was established by the Director of Food and Nutrition Services to evaluate the problem and recommend solutions. The group began by carefully defining the problem they were convened to address. The performance improvement (PI) coordinator insisted the problem be very specifically defined to keep the group focused. The following opportunity statement was developed: "An opportunity exists to streamline the process of ordering, preparing, and delivering patient late trays, beginning with the nurse's decision and ending with delivery of the meal to the patient." The principal customers were defined as patients, nurses, unit secretaries, PCTs, diet clerks, and food service assistants.

Once there was consensus on the opportunity statement, the next challenge was to define the current process for late tray delivery. Every member of the team understood the late tray process from his or her point of view. Our PI coordinator suggested we draw a flow diagram describing the process (Figure 1). Team members were amazed at the number of steps and complexity of what seemed to have been a very simple process. There were eighteen steps and seven different people involved in providing a late tray meal to a patient.

The next step was to collect data in order to further define the process and to begin to describe, with data, possible areas to focus our efforts. A time study was done to describe elapsed time between each of the eighteen steps. We learned that the average time from Step 1 (nurse determines patient needs a tray) to Step 18 (patient receives a tray) was eighty-one minutes.

A simple survey was distributed to the PCTs asking how long they were away from the floor to retrieve late trays, and what suggestions they had to make the process more efficient. The PCT returned completed surveys to the cashier in the cafeteria in exchange for a free freshly baked cookie. Results indicated PCTs were away from the floor from two to thirty minutes with the majority being away between five and ten minutes. There were a number of creative suggestions for improvement, and these were shared with the team.

The PI team participated in a brainstorming session led by the PI coordinator. The purpose was to identify all possible causes for late trays. Once the brainstorming session was complete, the ideas were organized into an Ishikawa (fishbone) diagram (Figure 2). Causes were grouped in like categories including Education, Systems, Communication, Materials, and Process.

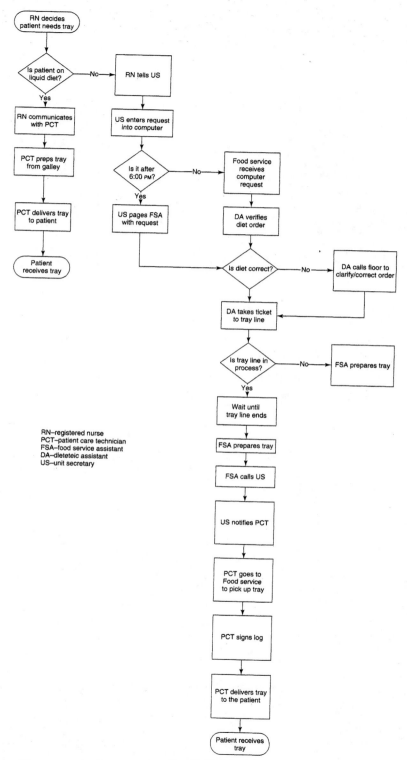

RN decides patient needs tray

Is patient on liquid diet? —No→ RN tells US

Yes

RN communicates with PCT

US enters request into computer

PCT preps tray from galley

Is it after 6:00 PM? —No→ Food service receives computer request

PCT delivers tray to patient

Yes

US pages FSA with request

DA verifies diet order

Patient receives tray

Is diet correct? —No→ DA calls floor to clarify/correct order

DA takes ticket to tray line

Is tray line in process? —No→ FSA prepares tray

Yes

Wait until tray line ends

FSA prepares tray

RN–registered nurse
PCT–patient care technician
FSA–food service assistant
DA–dieteteic assistant
US–unit secretary

FSA calls US

US notifies PCT

PCT goes to Food service to pick up tray

PCT signs log

PCT delivers tray to the patient

Patient receives tray

Figure 1   Late Tray PI Team Original Process

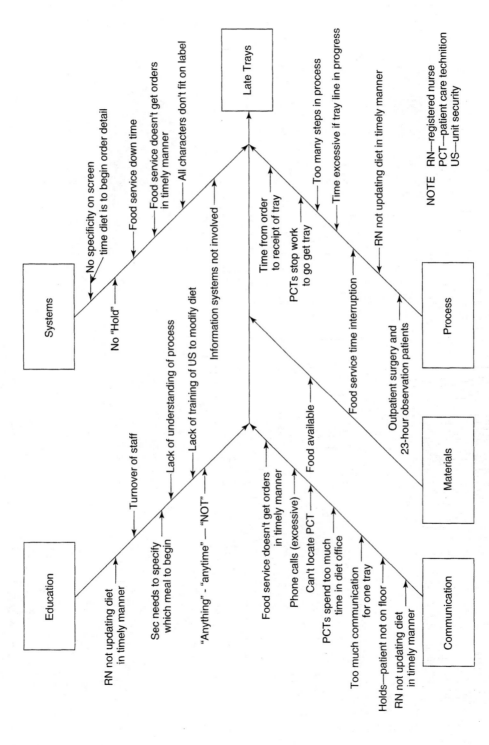

Figure 4–2 Late Tray PI Team: Brainstorming

The team used the fishbone diagram to determine other data that needed to be collected to validate some of the causes for late trays and to better understand the current process. A review of the literature was also done to learn how other institutions might have addressed the same problem.

The next step in the process was to begin to identify potential solutions. There was consensus that there were too many steps, too many people, and ineffective communication complicating the process. The team participated in another brainstorming session to identify possible solutions.

The new and improved late tray process was reduced from eighteen to seven steps (Figure 3 on page 62). The number of people involved in the process went from seven to four, and the average elapsed time was reduced from eighty-one minutes to fifteen minutes. The solution involved the nurse communicating directly with the PCT, who was no longer required to have the unit secretary enter an order in the computer, which had to be processed by the diet clerk. The PCT went directly to the kitchen and spoke with the food service assistant, signed a meal pick-up form, and delivered the late "meal to go" directly to the patient.

The solution was implemented, and a follow-up evaluation was conducted to evaluate whether the improvement was truly an improvement. The results indicated that improvements were sustained. As part of the brainstorming solutions session, an idea emerged to eliminate late tray service and provide "room service" for all patient meals. The obvious next step was to establish a new PI team and the process continued.

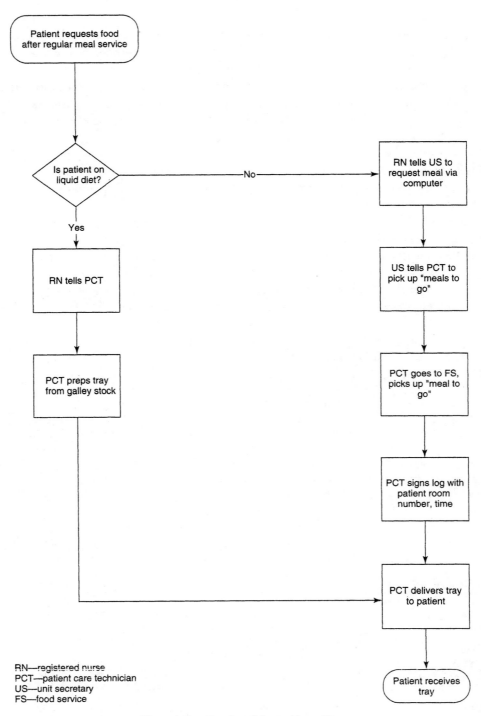

Patient requests food
after regular meal service

Is patient on
liquid diet?

No

RN tells US to
request meal via
computer

Yes

RN tells PCT

US tells PCT to
pick up "meals to
go"

PCT preps tray
from galley stock

PCT goes to FS,
picks up "meal to
go"

PCT signs log with
patient room
number, time

PCT delivers tray
to patient

RN—registered nurse
PCT—patient care technician
US—unit secretary
FS—food service

Patient receives
tray

Figure 3   Revised Late Tray Flow

62

Questions

1. Who might you assemble to serve on the performance improvement team to address the late tray problem?
2. What ideas for solving this problem might you expect to emerge in the brain-storming session?
3. How was the flow chart used in the PI process described?
4. What is the purpose of the Ishikawa (fishbone) diagram?
5. Why was it important to have a diverse team?
6. Describe the steps in the PI process used in this example.

Implementing Room Service in the Hospital

Objectives

At the completion of this case study, students should be able to:

1. Identify the benefits of room service compared to traditional hospital food service delivery systems.
2. Describe the need to have a multidisciplinary team in process improvement.
3. Describe challenges associated with major systems changes.

Case Narrative

A performance improvement (PI) team was established to improve the process for delivery of food to patients in an acute care hospital setting. The initial focus of the team was to address the number of late trays required by patients who were not available for meals at the regularly scheduled meal delivery period. One of the recommended solutions was to implement room service as a delivery model for all patient food service.

Traditional patient meal service involves the Food Services department preparing and delivering meals to patients at designated times for breakfast, lunch, dinner, and snack. Patients may select from a menu in advance, order from a spoken menu, or have preselected foods delivered from a cycle menu with consideration for their food preferences. They have little control over what or when they eat.

Meal schedules are determined collaboratively by Nursing and Food Services and occur on a rotation until all patients receive a meal. The challenges inherent in this system are numerous. Patients' shortened length of stay and increased acuity add to the complexity of the task. Patients are moved from place to place within the building as their health status changes. Many systems within the Food Services department are not sensitive enough to react quickly when many patients transfer from one room to another. A significant number of meals are wasted due to patient transfers.

Patient diet orders also change frequently. Diet changes result in a lot of waste when patients whose doctors have ordered that they not be given food by mouth (NPO) receive meals in error, and patient dissatisfaction occurs when patients are told they may eat and there is no meal for them when the trays are delivered. These issues also create a significant amount of work for and dissatisfaction within the Nursing department and cause increases in their workload.

The rising cost of healthcare is a concern for everyone in the industry. It is the responsibility of every hospital employee and department to identify ways to be more fiscally responsible. The amount of food wasted, an unnecessary cost, was evident with the traditional method of food service delivery. Also, the labor associated with the delivery of late trays was a concern. These issues and the opportunity to improve patient satisfaction with food services led us to initiate another PI team.

In February of 1998 a PI team was established to explore the concept of room service. The team included representatives from the nursing, clinical nutrition, food service management, performance improvement, rehabilitation services, information services, finance, and facilities departments. The team used a PI model to address the concept.

The first step was to do a review of the literature to identify other healthcare institutions using room service. The search yielded few results. We learned about St. Charles Medical Center in Bend, Oregon, which renovated its kitchen and was providing patient snacks and floor stock supplies via room service. A core group from the team (two nurses, one registered dietitian, one food service manager) made a site visit. The registered dietitian and food service manager also visited Brigham and Women's Hospital and LaHey Clinic in Boston, Massachusetts. These two facilities began to offer room service in partnership with Sodexho, a contract management company.

Room service eliminates scheduled mealtimes. Much like room service in the hotel industry, hospital room service allows patients to call and order what they want when they want it. Menus are maintained in each patient room. The housekeeping staff ensures that when a room is cleaned after a patient is discharged, a menu is available for the next patient admitted. The menu was designed with a variety of diet types in mind. There is also a note at the bottom of the menu indicating that due to the diet ordered by the patient's physician, some menu items may not be allowed.

Patients are oriented to the room service concept by the Nursing department personnel upon admission. The menu, system for ordering, and phone number to call for service are provided for the patients. If they are too ill or are otherwise unable to order for themselves, there are several options. Family members or the nursing staff may assist, or the Food Services department can place the patient on a menu schedule. The latter option was discouraged in an effort to give the patient and family more choices about when and what the patient eats.

The goals for implementing room service were to reduce waste in food, reduce labor associated with late tray delivery, reduce the amount of food stocked on patient care units (most of which was being consumed by staff), and improve patient satisfaction. Another primary driver for the project was space. Each nursing unit had a large galley, a food service area that had been used in the past to support a cook–freeze food delivery system. The hospital was undergoing a major automation initiative and identified the galley as space that could be converted to meet the automation needs.

The PI team worked together to design the new system, develop communication tools to educate the entire hospital staff, and create an implementation plan. Room service affected many departments and processes throughout the institution. A change of this magnitude required approval all the way up to the board of directors. The team had a challenge convincing many people that the change would be good for the patients and the institution. They earned approval, and room service began in November 1999.

The team made the decision to "go live" throughout the hospital as opposed to conducting a pilot program. The decision was made based on how difficult it would be for the food service staff to maintain parallel delivery systems that were so different. In preparation for the "go-live" date, the food service staff practiced by having nursing staff members order their meals via room service. They operated from a small makeshift area set up in the food production area. This strategy proved effective because the nurses were able to order a free meal and provide feedback about the service, food, and process while the food services staff practiced.

Room service required the addition of a new computer system and minor facility renovations. A touchscreen computer system was installed in the diet office to facilitate taking orders and communicating with the food production areas. The diet office and production staff had to learn the new system. The tray assembly line was converted to workspace, and a room service assembly area was relocated closer to the cold and hot food production areas. New patient food carts for meal delivery were ordered. The new carts held fewer trays to reduce delays caused by the temptation to fill up a cart before beginning delivery. A commitment was made to patients that they would receive their food within forty-five minutes of placing an order.

The start-up cost of $134,800 for room service included the following expenses:

$15,000 consulting fees

$18,000 computer system

$12,800 capital/construction

$89,000 incremental annual cost for food service labor.

The room service program saved $28,900 in reallocated space for the computer project and $88,000 in annual food cost, a savings of $116,900. While the room service net cost was $17,900, the nursing department was able to reassign 7.3 nursing FTEs to clinical tasks, as opposed to food service-related tasks, which resulted in greater job satisfaction.

The PI team conducted a number of quality measures to evaluate the effectiveness of the room service program. A staff satisfaction survey was administered three months after implementation. The staff responses indicated a 93 percent overall satisfaction rating with the program. Patient satisfaction improved by 12 percent overall. Patients were asked to evaluate taste, temperature, quality, appearance, variety, accuracy, and service. A significant improvement was noted in every category.

The time required for patients to receive meals improved from 81 minutes to between 19 and 21 minutes. Patients were able to get the food they wanted in significantly less time than it had taken prior to the conversion. Tray waste studies in the dishwashing area indicated a significant reduction in trays returned with food uneaten.

Some of the outcomes that were unexpected included the satisfaction expressed by the food service staff. The pace of work and peak times changed, and the dishwashing room became a much less chaotic area because the dirty dishes did not all come to the kitchen at the same time for cleaning and return to service. The dishwashing staff made regular rounds throughout all the patient floors on their time schedule and washed dishes throughout the day.

The hospital had an opportunity to use the new system as a marketing opportunity. The project was featured both internally and within the community as a means of providing patient-centered care. It was cited as an example of interdisciplinary performance improvement during the 2000 survey by the Joint Commission for Accreditation of Healthcare Organizations. The room service program assisted our hospital in meeting its mission of taking the best care of every patient every day.

Questions

1. What are the advantages of room service compared to traditional hospital food service?
2. What is the benefit of having a variety of disciplines participate on the PI team?
3. What considerations are important when implementing major systems changes?

Cases in Safety and Sanitation

THE CEILING IS FALLING!

THE CAFETERIA SERVER WITH A NOSE RING

LONG-TERM CARE MOCK SURVEY: KITCHEN SANITATION INSPECTION

The Ceiling Is Falling!

Objectives

At the completion of this case study, students should be able to:

1. Recognize that the careful monitoring of employees is necessary, especially when you are not familiar with their level of judgment and abilities.
2. Make a quick and thorough assessment of a situation, remain calm, and take action.

Case Narrative

While Marcia was in college, one undergraduate degree program provided her with the opportunity to manage one of the university's restaurants in the student union. She had spent time before the rotation planning the menu, work schedule, and purchasing plan. This was all then approved by her instructor, who was also the manager of the cafeteria.

She was nervous as the week started. Things went fine for breakfast and lunch that first day, and she breathed a sigh of relief. In the afternoon, pots were stewing, dishes were being done, and salads were being prepared. Everything looked fine.

Unbeknownst to her, however, trouble was brewing. Paul, a hospitality student who was cleaning pots and pans, was having great difficulty separating two large eight- to ten-gallon pots that had been stacked inside one another. To get them apart he placed them on the stove and turned the flame to high. Then he returned to the sink and washed a few more items.

After five or ten minutes, the pans started making a noise. Paul went to see if he could pull them apart. As he approached the stove, the top pot shot up into the ceiling, shooting steam all over and into his eyes. Part of the ceiling fell out. He screamed and fell to the ground with his hands over his eyes. As Marcia was running over, a manager from the nearby cafeteria ran in. She quickly assessed the situation, yelled, "Call 911!" and began to assist the young man on the floor. At this point, Paul was going into shock; someone brought blankets to cover him up. The paramedics came, stabilized their patient, and took him to the hospital. The area was cleaned up, and dinner proceeded.

The next day, Marcia learned that Paul's eyes had been burned and that he would need to be in complete darkness for three days, but his vision would not be harmed. The ceiling would take a few weeks to repair. Incident reports and forms needed to be filed. Marcia went over this whole incident in her head so many times that she was glad when the week was over.

Questions

1. How could Paul have separated the pots?
2. When should you call 911? If you're not sure, should you do it to be on the safe side?

The Cafeteria Server with a Nose Ring

Objectives

At the completion of this case study, students should be able to:

1. Balance humanitarian causes with good business and sanitation principles.
2. Identify some sanitation hazards and take effective steps to eliminate them.
3. Recognize that consumers are concerned about sanitation.

Case Narrative

Helen is a nurse in a medium-sized urban hospital in Los Angeles. She decided to eat in the hospital cafeteria one day. As she arrived in the cafeteria and was approaching the counter, she observed the employee behind the counter combing her long black hair with her fingers. The employee saw Helen and straightened up, adjusting her nose ring in the process.

"Are you ready?" she asked.

"No, thank you," Helen hastily replied as she headed toward the vending machines. She picked up a comment card on her way. While she was eating, Helen filled out the comment card, which was addressed to the hospital administrator. She explained on the comment card her revulsion at the server's nose ring and sanitation habits. She dropped it in the box on her way back to the nursing unit.

About three days later, Helen received a call from the food service director. He was genuinely concerned. He revealed to Helen that this particular employee is a troubled teen to whom he had been trying to give an extra chance. She had since been fired for lack of improvement.

73

Questions

1. What other ways could the food service director have found to give this employee an extra chance?
2. Is the nose ring truly a problem? If so, why?
3. Could you legally deny employment to a person with a nose ring?
4. What other behavior of the serving employee was undesirable?

Long-Term Care Mock Survey

Kitchen Sanitation Inspection

Objectives

Upon completion of this case study, students should be able to:

1. Identify food safety hazards in a food service operation.
2. Prioritize food safety concerns based on the potential to cause food-borne illness.
3. Work with dietary supervisors and staff to develop and implement a plan of correction.

Case Narrative

Don has been selected by his nursing home company to join a multidisciplinary team for a mock Department of Health survey of a nearby nursing facility. As a food service director, he will be responsible for inspecting the dietary department.

On the day of the survey, he enters the kitchen unannounced at 9:30 A.M. To his right a food service employee is slicing meats for sandwiches. Several hams, turkeys, and cheeses are on a cart near him. There are some scraps of ham on the table around the slicer. The sliced meat is stacked in several clean pans.

On Don's left he notices the three-compartment pot-washing sink. There are chicken legs floating loose in warm water in the last compartment on the right. The supervisor reports that the chicken was frozen and is now being defrosted for lunch.

The walls and ceiling look clean, but there is dust on the ceiling air vents and sprinkler heads. There are crumbs on the floor around the toaster. Don hears staff members take calls and fill requests from the nursing floors for late breakfast trays.

In the storeroom, an employee is putting away the food order. Many stacks of cases fill the room. The frozen and refrigerated food is piled nearest to the door where he is standing. The employee is moving new whole cases of condiments and canned foods onto the storeroom shelves. He says this is a good way to have the date received marked on the food.

The cook is slicing potatoes for potato salad. She sneezes occasionally, but then washes her hands thoroughly and returns to her task. A check of the kitchen hand-washing sink reveals potato scrapings in the bottom; only cold water is available, and the soap dispenser is empty.

Questions

1. Which problems did Don see that could result in a food-borne illness?
2. Do the scraps of lunchmeat around the slicer and the crumbs on the floor near the toaster pose a major, moderate, or minor food safety risk? Explain.
3. What are two ways the food order could have been put away more safely?
4. List at least two departmental policies, procedures, or other actions that would decrease the food safety risk to the nursing home residents.

General References

Grossbauer, S. 2002. *Managing Foodservice Operations: A Systems Approach for Healthcare and Institutions.* 4th ed. Dubuque, Iowa: Kendall-Hunt.

U.S. Public Health Service, Food and Drug Administration. 1999. *Food Code.* Washington, D.C.: U.S. Department of Health and Human Services.

Internet References

Partnership for Food Safety Education
www.fightbac.org
National Restaurant Association Educational Foundation
www.edfound.org
Dietary Managers Association
www.dmaonline.org

Cases in Management of Food Services

THEFT OPPORTUNITY: WHO DID IT?

FOOD SERVICE PLAN DURING A STRIKE

CHANGING FROM CONTRACT TO SELF-OPERATED
AND BACK AGAIN

BALANCING WORK AND FAMILY: WHEN CHILDCARE
COLLIDES WITH WORK EXPECTATIONS

TOO SICK, TOO SOON!

Theft Opportunity

Who Did It?

Objectives

At the completion of this case study, students should be able to:

1. Evaluate ease of access into and out of storage areas and facilities.
2. Evaluate standing policies and procedures and enforcement of such policies for routine delivery times.
3. Evaluate employee schedules for periods of time when one or two employees are alone in the department.
4. Evaluate the need for camera surveillance based upon the layout and design of the department.

Case Narrative

Theft is a serious concern in food service operations as in any business. This theft opportunity took place in the dietary department housed in a school for people with special needs. The department is open Monday through Friday year round. The dietary department hours are routinely from 6:00 A.M. to 2:30 P.M. for food production, service, and clean-up activities. The kitchen manager, dietitian, and secretary work eight hours per day from 8:00 A.M. to 4:30 P.M. and are located in an office next to the kitchen. The department produces approximately 150 breakfasts and 650 lunches per day of operation. The manager, dietitian, secretary, head cook, head of the night custodian service, three maintenance workers, and the administrator have keys to the dietary department office and kitchen. Once the kitchen is unlocked in the morning at 6:00 A.M., all kitchen doors and storage areas

79

remain unlocked throughout the day until 2:30 P.M., when the last of the kitchen workers leave. Sometime between 2:30 P.M. and 3:00 P.M., the manager would do the final walk-through to check the kitchen and lock all doors and storage areas. The office door is not locked until 4:30 P.M. The office has an internal door access into the kitchen that is never locked.

The cooking staff is scheduled to work staggered shifts beginning, with the first cook arriving at 6:00 A.M. and the dishroom workers and potwashers arriving last at 8:00 A.M. All kitchen staff are expected to be present for the lunch meal service, which is scheduled from 11:00 A.M. to 12:45 P.M. Because of the special population served, the dietary department staffs three separate lunch serving sites within the school. The full-time kitchen staff works 6½ hours per day. The part-time kitchen staff usually works a maximum of 4 hours per day. The cooking staff is responsible for cooking, baking, serving, and cleaning activities. The aides are responsible for delivering breakfast foods and snacks to classrooms, preportioning food items, serving food at lunch, and cleaning activities. The dishroom workers and potwashers are responsible for washing the baker's and cooks' pots and pans; washing lunch dishes; replenishing tray lines with clean dishes, trays, and so on throughout the lunch service time; and sweeping and mopping the department floors, with the exception of the large cafeteria floor. The large cafeteria floor is done at night by the night custodian service that is responsible for all of the floors throughout the school.

The lead cook or manager checks in the morning food deliveries. The manager or, occasionally, the dietitian or the secretary checks in the afternoon food deliveries. Food deliveries of milk and ice cream always arrive at 6:00 A.M. Produce deliveries routinely arrive by 8:30 A.M. The large food deliveries of all other items, including chemicals and paper goods, routinely come on Mondays and Thursdays in the afternoon between 2:00 P.M. and 3:00 P.M. Recently, however, the delivery times for the large food deliveries had been changing. The truck drivers were now frequently arriving during the lunch service time. Although the manager fussed at the drivers for their poor timing, she continued to accept their deliveries and she put away the frozen and refrigerated stock during the lunch meal service time. The manager would then leave the rest of the delivery on the floor in the back hallway outside of the dry goods storeroom until she could get back to it later that afternoon. This back hallway is where the drivers stacked all their items as they brought them in from the trucks.

The delivery back door is within 15 feet of the dry goods storage room and the main walk-in freezer and refrigerator. Large and small trucks and other vehicles can back up to within 8 feet of the kitchen delivery door. There is no loading dock at this delivery door. The delivery door is just off a large employee parking area that is shared between the school and a large medical center. The parking area is very active, with people coming and going throughout the day and night. Two very active side streets border the parking area. Street parking is also allowed on both sides of one of these streets.

Kitchen staffing had been changing over the past several months. Several long-term employees had retired, two had transferred to other departments, and one had married and moved out of state. Although active recruiting was in progress, the shortage of kitchen staff was at a crisis level. Through the recruiting and interviewing process, only one aide had been hired. The decision was made to seek temporary employees from a local temp agency and to continue the recruiting efforts. Within the week the temp agency sent a cook, an aide, and two dishwashers. All four temporary employees learned their jobs quickly and settled into the kitchen routine without incident.

Because of illness, jury duty, and unavoidable scheduled days off, the kitchen was still short the number of employees needed for normal operations, so the manager, secretary, and dietitian continued to assist with lunch service. When truck deliveries arrived at lunchtime, the manager would direct the truck driver to work with either the cook replenishing the pans of food for service lines or one of the dishroom workers if the cook was busy. The cook or the dishroom worker would check in the delivery and have the frozen stock stacked on the floor of the freezer, the cold stock stacked on the floor of the refrigerator, and everything else stacked in the back hallway. After lunch service was completed, the manager would sort and store all of the delivery items in the appropriate storage areas.

Within two weeks, the manager and the cooks started noticing missing items. At first it was a few cases of frozen meat and then it grew to frozen meats, cooler items, and cases of vegetables. The invoices indicated that the missing cases were received, but when the cooks went to pull the menu item for cooking, one or more cases or cans would be missing. One afternoon, all of the cases of special steaks that had been ordered for an important school board meeting were discovered missing within two hours of their arrival to the kitchen.

The manager estimated that the thefts had cost her department more than $17,000 in food by the time the thefts were solved and stopped.

Questions

1. Were the kitchen and storage areas easily accessed? Explain your answer.
2. How could the kitchen and storage area access be limited without interfering with kitchen operations?
3. Did the change in the delivery time by the truckers provide opportunity for theft to occur? Explain your answer.
4. How could the manager and dietitian use the department's employee schedules to eliminate suspects?
5. Would camera surveillance with tape recording capability help prevent this type of theft in the future?

Food Service Plan During a Strike

Objectives

At the completion of this case study, students should be able to:

1. Describe some of the challenges that a manager faces when a work force strikes.
2. Identify several strategies for coping with an employee strike.
3. Complete a schedule and a plan for feeding staff and patients while union employees are on strike.

Case Narrative

A labor dispute was brewing at Broadworth Community Hospital, a 140-bed general medical center. Broadworth's food service department includes a food service director, four dietitians, an outpatient dietitian, two per diem dietitians, two certified dietary managers, and thirty full-time equivalents (FTEs) of hourly workers. It is an independently managed food service. The hospital is responsible for the food service to the patients as well as the staff. There are approximately five hundred hospital staff members and some visitors who dine in the cafeteria Monday through Friday for breakfast and lunch. There is a busy catering schedule for various meetings and educational programs. Approximately 25 percent of the food is prepared from scratch. The cooks roast their own beef and turkeys and make their own stews. Soups and puddings are canned.

The cafeteria features three entrées along with vegetables, salads, and desserts. The patient menus include regular, soft, pureed, mechanical soft, low-residue, clear liquid, full liquid, diabetic, renal, renal diabetic, weight reduction,

82

low-salt, low-cholesterol, and low-fat diets. Breakfast includes two hot cereals as well as cold cereals, two entrées, juice, fruit, and breakfast pastries. There is a selective menu for lunch and dinner that includes two entrées; two soups; and a variety of fruits, vegetables, and desserts with all the accessories to go with a well-balanced meal.

After a prolonged and ongoing labor dispute, the nonmanagerial employees at Broadworth voted to go on strike. When the strike was announced, the members of the food service management team were not surprised. They had anticipated the possibility and made preliminary plans but were still nervous. The hospital administrators communicated to the food service managers that the remaining employees would receive free meals while on duty for all three shifts, seven days a week. Once the strike began, the cafeteria patronage dropped to about one hundred employees, which included management, physicians, medical residents, temporary employees, and nursing staff. All catering was placed on hold. The food service department purchased food from a variety of purveyors. Some purveyors continued to deliver food on schedule; others, such as the bakery company, were unionized and would not cross the picket line.

Many of the hospital floors were closed. The physical rehabilitation floor, psychiatric floor, emergency room, and a limited number of beds were available for telemetry, intensive care, medical–surgical, and orthopedic patients. Before the strike started, many of the patients were discharged or transferred to a sister hospital or an acute care hospital. When the strike started, there were approximately thirty patients in the hospital.

All members of the management team were notified when the strike was called. The team finalized its strike plans and buckled down for the long haul. The strike lasted nearly a month, and everyone was relieved when it was finally resolved.

Questions

1. How can the food service operation be simplified to accommodate the strike by utilizing the small staff on hand?
2. How can the food service management use the remaining staff to best serve the patients and fellow employees? (The management team, dietitians, and approximately six temporary, nonunionized employees were available.)
3. What could the management team do to better prepare for the strike?

Changing from Contract to Self-Operated and Back Again

Objectives

At the completion of this case study, students should be able to:

1. Identify and list problems faced by new management teams.
2. Suggest detailed solutions to identified problems.
3. Understand and explain the relationship between a client and a food service manager.

Case Narrative

Pauline Herrera, administrator for the senior living center, prepared for her meeting with the food service director. She was reviewing information obtained from employee satisfaction surveys. The information apparently came from center employees who worked in the food service area managed by the contract food service company. The survey results indicated low morale, potential turnover, and general dissatisfaction by employees in that department. She wondered about the working conditions in the food service department. What could be done for these employees to improve their morale and prevent turnover? A bigger concern was the capability of the management company and whether awarding them the food service management contract had been a mistake.

This case was originally written as a result of a CHRIE Faculty Internship and used with the permission of International CHRIE.

Introduction

The food service management company, or contractor, was new to this account (nine months). The account was a senior living center operated as part of a large Catholic hospital, located just a block away. Prior to the arrival of the new contractor, the facility had been operated by a Jewish affiliated hospital. At that time, the hospital operated a kosher kitchen, and a rabbi was the overseer of food preparation. The center primarily catered to senior patients with rehabilitation needs and others with long-term illnesses. The change to the Catholic hospital affiliation and the hiring of the food service contractor had occurred in a nine-month period.

The food service at the hospital was self-operated and had a long and successful history. The food service director at the hospital had maintained that position for twenty years and was well respected in the community. Administrators for the hospital and the center were considering a change in the future that would coincide with the retirement of their long-term food service director. The senior living center was the test case for this experiment.

The center had fifty beds, and the food service department was responsible for providing meals to all patients three times per day, as well as a snack. These meals were prepared based on the dietary instructions of the doctors and nurses, working with the dietitian, an employee of the food service contractor. The food service operation also had a small retail outlet for center employees and visitors. The café, as it was referred to, provided a mixture of sandwiches, drinks, salads, and complete meals. The two most active times in this facility were lunch and breakfast, respectively. Finally, catering was a fast growing part of the food service business for the contractor. Catered events were anything from coffee and pastries for a breakfast staff meeting to sit-down, white tablecloth dinners for the board of directors. The development of this segment of the business required a strong marketing effort by the managers. To increase catering sales, the food service contractor needed to be flexible, quick to respond, and able to provide high-quality services and products. Inherently, this would mean a well-trained staff that could adjust and react to many situations quickly.

Current food service employees had extensive experience in this operation. They had worked for or with rabbis, nuns, independent food service directors, and other food service contractors. The new food service management team was composed of a director, an assistant director in charge of production, and a dietitian. All the other food service employees, including the diet technicians, were center employees. The hospital administrators were looking to the management company for high-quality products and services and, above all, their ability to save money.

The Employees

The fifteen employees in the food service department had a range of experience in the center from four to twenty-five years. The ages of employees ranged from their early twenties to late fifties, approximately half male and half female. Interaction between and among employees was positive. Everyone appeared to get along well.

Generally, food service employees were skeptical of food service management companies and their managers. They felt that the food service management contractors did not care about their employees and were only concerned with the bottom line. The hospital food service employees considered themselves lucky that they were not employed by the management company but were employees of the hospital. The center food service employees also felt that the food service contractor was interested only in the bottom line; as long as the contractor made money, it did not care what happened to the employees. The employees complained that since the food service contractor had taken over the account, they were constantly being asked to do more with less. They were also expected to be cross-trained and be able to perform any task. They felt that being asked to do more and learn more meant more responsibility without additional compensation. However, the food service employees were not unionized, and they felt helpless. They had seen staff cutbacks before and were leery that they might happen again. The fifteen food service employees were composed of three catering employees, three service employees who worked in the retail area provided for the center's employees, three food prep employees including dishwashers, three cooks, and three food-line workers.

The food service employees at the main hospital were also watching the food service contractor. They wondered whether many of their jobs would be eliminated if the hospital hired a food service contractor for the entire facility. The main hospital food service employees monitored the smaller facility by staying in touch with the senior living center employees on a regular basis.

The Management

In the short time the food service management company had been at the facility, the food service director, Ralph Martin, had developed a routine. He completed all the opening paperwork, reviewed the logbook for any special notices, and then dealt with the production scheduling for the day in conjunction with dietary staff. Mr. Martin then supervised the production line for breakfast trays to ensure that all patients received their meals in a timely manner and in accordance with their prescribed diet. He then visited all floors in the facility, spoke to the charge nurses on each floor, and randomly spoke with a number of patients to solicit input on items such as food quality and adherence to specifications. His morning walks through the center were much appreciated by the staff and the patients and made his job easier. His relationship with the hospital staff was excellent. However, the director did find that he had to mediate the relationships between the dietitian and the nursing staff. These interactions had been troublesome in the past and continued to be so. The crux of the issues appeared to be communication problems concerning patient meals and changes made from original instructions.

Ralph Martin was confronted with the information that Pauline Herrera had concerning employee morale in his department. Ralph realized that he had a serious problem. He had not been aware that the problem was this serious, although he knew some of the employees were unhappy with the change in management. He had worked hard to communicate with the center staff, and this seemed to be working. He speculated that a big part of the problem was that the employees were blaming him and the food service management company for labor cutbacks that were initiated after they took over the account. Prior to the food service company's coming on board there had been twenty-nine food service employees. The manager wanted to explain to the employees that the cuts in staffing were part of a package of money-saving ideas that the center administrators wanted and that these cuts would have been made whether it was their company that won the contract or not. Ralph believed that the reason a contract food service company was brought in was its ability to save money and that the employees needed to understand that.

Shortly after Ralph Martin arrived, he had conducted employee performance evaluations. Ralph had examined the skills and abilities of all the employees, their past records, and their current performance and decided that some changes needed to be made. In addition to the fourteen employees who were terminated, one employee had been demoted or reassigned because of his poor reading skills. Employees who had been used to doing things on their own found themselves following written and enforced standards and procedures and were not happy about it. Despite the changes that were made, managers did feel that to provide some of the additional services being requested by the hospital staff more employees were necessary.

Conclusion

Ralph Martin knew that he and the food service management company that he worked for had a real opportunity to expand the account and his own responsibilities. If he was successful and delivered high-quality food service with a trimmed staff, the food service company might get the entire hospital food service account when the hospital food service director retired. That would increase the size of the account, and it would put Ralph in line for a bigger job with more responsibility. These things probably would not happen with employee morale problems and a center administrator concerned about employee morale and turnover. Ralph knew that he would have to deal with these problems, but he was not sure just how to do it. What were the real issues here? The history of changes in management had placed Ralph in a tough situation. Were the issues communication, work environment, organizational change, team orientation, or company relations with the administrator? Was it a combination of all five? Ralph needed to act quickly and in a way that was responsive to the employees and the administration.

Questions

1. Why are employees at this facility concerned about the food service management company?
2. What are the roots of their concerns?
3. How can the manager alleviate these concerns?

Balancing Work and Family

When Childcare Collides with Work Expectations

Objectives

At the completion of this case study, students will be able to:

1. Clarify why a policy not permitting employees' children in the workplace exists.
2. Distinguish between an employee with good performance and the separate issue of not complying with the "no children at work" policy.
3. Consider options existing for employees to work and also comply with this policy rule.

Case Narrative

PM is an excellent female production manager who, when present, is fair and thorough and always motivates her employees to get the job done. In the past eight months, she has worked twelve-hour days to cover for supervisor shortages and assisted MR, the food service director, in developing, revising, and submitting the budget for the next fiscal year. The hospital has been considering PM for a promotion based on her performance and her excellent interpersonal skills.

As a single parent, PM has sole custody and responsibility for two school-age children, ages six and ten. She has no backup for when the children are sick and are unable to attend school. In the summer, a neighbor watches the children for a fee.

During the last two weeks PM's children have been on antibiotics for an infection; they were not allowed in school for forty-eight hours. PM brought each child to work several days and left the child in MR's office. MR was on vacation and did not find this out until yesterday. The facility and department rule is that no one can bring a sick child to work. The management does not allow any of the food service department employees to bring children to work.

Questions

1. Describe the problem MR faces.
2. Why can't the management change the rule and allow sick children to come to the facility?
3. What must be discussed with PM?
4. Determine what solutions or options exist.

Too Sick, Too Soon!

Objectives

At the completion of this case study, students should be able to:

1. Understand the qualifications for the Family and Medical Leave Act.
2. Examine the strength of the negotiated agreement, the supervisor's obligation to discipline, the progressive discipline process, and the human side of the issue.

Case Narrative

Backwater City Schools is a school district in Southwest Ohio just outside of Dayton. There are about 7,000 students enrolled in the district's eight schools. The food service department consists of full cooking kitchens in the high school and the two middle schools and finishing kitchens in the five elementary schools. The food service is self-operated. The annual budget is about $1.6 million. There are about fifty employees in the food service department, but half of them work fewer than three hours per day due to the configuration of a modified base–satellite system. At the elementary schools the employees are basically there only to serve the meal and clean up afterward. The pay is good—entry-level employees make $11.50 an hour with no specialized training required—but the paychecks are still very small. Some of the servers work only two hours per day, so it is not a lot of money for the commitment of being available each day at lunchtime. Also, a fee of $200 per year is taken out for union dues from these hourly employees. Finding just the right employees for school food service

91

is a constant challenge. There are a lot of good things about never having to work weekends and being off in the summer, but if you really need to work you probably can't afford the luxury of a two-hour-a-day job! And it takes more than five years to work up to a full-time job with the system. However, those full-time positions are still only six hours a day for less than 200 days, including paid holidays, so it never becomes a self-supporting career. The food service employees are covered by the agreement negotiated by the Backwater Classified Employees Association (BCEA). The document is fairly comprehensive, going into detail about the types of leave that employees can take. As soon as employees are hired, they receive 3 personal days and begin to accumulate sick leave at the rate of 1.5 days per month

Current Situation

Amy was hired in the spring for a 2.25-hour job at one of the middle schools. She was turning into an excellent employee, proficient at the cash register and at serving. Over the summer, she began to have back problems. She tried to return to work, but some days the pain was too bad. She was under a doctor's care, and the doctor said that she needed to take some time off from work so her back could heal. Amy followed the doctor's orders, but soon she had exhausted all the sick leave she had earned during her short tenure with the district. After reading the negotiated agreement, she felt she could apply for five days' medical leave without pay.

Her supervisor approved the leave without pay, attaching the doctor's order for time off to the form. Two days later the leave form arrived back on the supervisor's desk marked "DENIED." The director of business had written a note on the form saying that this leave was not intended for short-term illnesses, but for major medical problems that would require an employee to miss work for an extended period of time. He suggested that she file for family and medical leave.

The supervisor knew that Amy did not legally qualify for leave under the Family and Medical Leave Act. She sent a note back to the director of business explaining that this was not an option for Amy and asked whether he had any suggestions as to how to cover these days, which Amy had already taken per her doctor's orders.

The director of business replied with this typed memo:

> If she has no leave authorization available, then this is an "absence without authority," a disciplinary matter. You need to give her a letter of warning advising that it is her responsibility to be at work or have some approved authorization to be absent. Furthermore, she needs to understand that if this is repeated, additional discipline will be necessary and that, ultimately, it may lead to her losing her job.

So, the supervisor started the disciplinary action against this good employee with the following letter:

October 18, 2002

To: Amy Smith, 2.25 hours @ AMS

From: Joyce Roberts
       Supervisor of Food Service

It has been brought to my attention that you did not qualify for the medical leave of five days that you requested and I approved. Since you had no leave available and there is no provision in our organization to cover your circumstance of being under a doctor's care and unable to work—even without pay—I need to inform you that this absence is considered being *absent without authority* even though we spoke often during this process.

I was incorrect in my thinking that you could write a letter and request permission to be off work as the doctor had ordered. I am sorry that I misled you. It is now my unpleasant duty to inform you that being absent without authority is considered a disciplinary matter, and you need to know that by my writing this letter you have been given a *written warning*. This warning is to inform you that further days off without a leave will result in disciplinary action. Through due process, the end result could be termination of your employment with Backwater City Schools.

I know you have struggled to balance your healing with your available sick leave. Since you are a new employee to our district, perhaps you may want to consider severing your employment with us on your terms, so there is no termination on your record. After your healing is complete, I would be happy to have you on the sub list if you wish to start over at the bottom again. What I do not want is for you to work with an injury just to keep this job. Your health is worth much more than this part-time job.

Just so you understand—if you miss another day's work before you have earned a sick day to cover that absence, I must continue the disciplinary process.

I acknowledge receipt of this letter and understand that a copy of it will be placed in my personnel file.

X _____   _____

SIGNATURE   DATE

Before the employee was able to return the letter, she called from the hospital where she had been admitted for a kidney stone. She had difficulty passing the stone and was hospitalized for three days. She returned to work with a note from her doctor stating that she had been in the hospital.

Questions

1. Why was the employee unable to apply for family and medical leave?

2. What do you think of the supervisor's letter? Is this how a written warning should sound?

3. Is discipline in order here?

4. Will discipline modify this employee's behavior?

5. Was this second absence allowable?

6. What should the supervisor do?

7. While there were several possible outcomes, the option the director of business chose was surprising. He struck a compromise. If Amy would agree to take the written warning in her personnel file (and she really had no choice in this matter), he would allow all the days missed up to this point to be considered as one occurrence and the warning letter would cover all those days—even though the first warning letter did not include the three days for the kidney stone. However, the next time she was absent—for whatever reason—before she had earned more sick leave, she would get three days off without pay, the next step in the discipline process. The next violation would result in termination. What do you think of this approach?

Cases in Nutrition Management

ISSUES WITH PRODUCTIVITY AND SALARY COMPLAINTS

CLINICAL MANAGEMENT: SEEING THE "BIG PICTURE"

DEALING WITH MANAGEMENT'S REQUEST TO REDUCE STAFFING

MARKETING OUTPATIENT NUTRITION COUNSELING

INAPPROPRIATE EMPLOYEE SELF-TERMINATION

Issues with Productivity and Salary Complaints

Objectives

At the completion of this case study, students should be able to:

1. Identify the need to research the validity of any second-hand information provided by subordinates on peers.
2. Define one professional approach to dealing with issues of productivity.
3. Determine the need to follow the chain of command.

Case Narrative

This case takes place in a 400-bed hospital that has four dietetic technicians (two full-time and two part-time) and two registered dietitians (RDs). There are two technicians scheduled every day, and the dietitians work Monday through Friday and are on call over the weekends. The dietitians have home access to the hospital computer system, enabling them to access a patient's laboratory results if necessary.

The job responsibilities for the dietetic technicians are as follows:

1. Print reports from the computer including a daily list of all patients, and a daily list of patients on all diets, including no food by mouth (NPO), clear or full liquids, and tube feedings by 7:00 A.M. From this information they prioritize patients to be seen by the RD or a technician by 8:00 A.M. when the dietitians arrive.

2. Review all nursing admission databases that contain "nutrition screens" on select units that have high illness (high acuity) levels. (While nursing is responsible for sending screening information to the dietary department on the high-turnover units, decreased nursing staffing has resulted in less information being sent to the dietary department.)
3. Offer basic diet instructions, including cardiac, low-residue, high-residue, and several other basic instructions under the supervision of the RDs. The RDs countersign all instruction notes in the chart.
4. Gather data for the RDs on patient flow forms for high-risk patients on total parenteral nutrition (TPN). This information is relayed to dietitians on weekends via computer from 9:00 A.M. to 10:00 A.M. for the RDs to review and contact nursing units with verbal recommendations for any changes to be made.

The job responsibilities for the dietitians, including all registered dietitians, are as follows:

1. Review the diet technicians' prioritization of patients each morning and countersign diet instructions on medical record sheets, which are either put in the chart or sent to medical records if the patient was discharged the day before.
2. Complete assessments on high-risk patients. Reassign patients found to be low functioning to the technicians.
3. See all high-risk patients and do all complex diet instructions such as those for diabetic and high calorie/protein diets.
4. On weekends, review computer information from 9:00 A.M. to 10:00 A.M. daily to determine any changes necessary in TPN or high-risk tube feedings. Any changes are called in to nursing units. Dietitians accrue one hour of comp time for every hour spent working on weekends.

History and type of staffing

Originally the hospital had 3½ dietitians with an average cost of $20 per hour (excluding benefits). As turnover occurred, the facility hired graduates of four-year dietetic programs as full-time technicians and third- and fourth-year dietetic students as part-time technicians. The technicians were paid an average of $10 per hour (excluding benefits), and only full-time employees were eligible for benefits. Two 8-hour technicians work Monday through Friday. On weekends, one 8-hour technician and one 4-hour technician work due to the lower census count. With the new system there has been less turnover in full-time positions, and the administration was pleased with the reduced costs of recruiting as well the reduced cost of agency dietitians. The staff believes patient care has improved.

Question

You are the director of patient food services at the hospital. You are faced with the following situations:

a. The newest part-time (20-hour-per-week) technician, RCM, never seems to get her work done. The quality of the work is adequate, but she gets 30 percent less work done than her coworkers, and her coworkers are complaining to you that she doesn't do her share of the work. RCM has successfully gone through your standard orientation and training program. To complicate matters, it has been reported to you that she has been observed having long, detailed conversations with a new medical resident in the intensive care unit, which is a unit she is not responsible for.

b. RCM is also not happy with her salary. While she reports directly to you, she has gone to see your supervisor, the food service director, twice. Each time he has told her to talk to you. Although she is only a third-year dietetics major, she believes she should earn the same amount per hour that your most senior technician (a four-year graduate who has worked for you for two years) is making because this is the amount she was told her college classmate is making at another hospital on the other side of the city.

How should you handle RCM and the concerns regarding (a) productivity and (b) salary?

Clinical Management

Seeing the "Big Picture"

Objectives

At the completion of this case study, students should be able to:

1. Identify how the hospital client for a contract food service company impacts decisions made in a dietary department.
2. Define how clinical dietitian behavior can positively and negatively impact hospital client decision making.
3. Determine approaches to assist the clinical dietitians in seeing the "big picture."

Case Narrative

The hospital is a 600-bed university teaching hospital that has contracted out the food service and the dietary department to a national contract food service company to control or reduce hospital food costs. Within the hospital, the director of the food service department (FSD), who is a registered dietitian employed by the contract company, answers to and is supervised by the vice president for ancillary services. Any decisions regarding budget must be submitted by the FSD both to the vice president and to the contract company regional operations director for approval.

The department has eight registered general practice clinical registered dietitians (RDs) and one RD nutrition support specialist. The dietitians answer to the clinical nutrition manager (CNM), who is also an RD. The CNM manages the diet office staff, the tray line staff, and the dietitians and answers to the FSD. The vice

100

president has told both the FSD and the CNM that his major concern for their department is food service—both food quality and how it is served to the patients. He has repeatedly indicated he is not interested in adding clinical registered dietitian staff. In fact, he has also commented that he has observed the clinical dietitians on inpatient units. The dietitians were not aware of his presence since they have not yet realized he is "the client" for the food service company. The limited interactions he has had with the clinical dietitians have left him unimpressed; he complained of their immaturity and inappropriate comments. He actually said he was glad they answered to food service and not to someone else (like him) within the hospital.

The clinical dietitians had concerns of their own. Last week the clinical dietitians contacted the regional dietitian for the contract company and asked for a meeting. In the meeting they said they were dissatisfied with the FSD and CNM, who were not meeting their needs. They told the regional dietitian they no longer wanted to visit patients during meals to assess whether they were eating and liked the food. Furthermore, they felt they needed two more clinical dietitians to ensure that they could get their work done, take an hour lunch, and keep up with their clinical reading in 8½ hours.

Questions

1. What conflict exists between the goals of the hospital client (the vice president) and the goals of the clinical dietitians? How can the conflict be addressed and/or resolved?

2. Did the clinical dietitians handle their concerns appropriately? Are these concerns legitimate?

3. Determine at least one way to assist the clinical dietitians in seeing the "big picture."

4. How might the CNM address some of the concerns associated with the behavior of the dietitians?

Dealing with Management's Request to Reduce Staffing

Objectives

At the completion of this case study, students should be able to:

1. Describe the political factors that must be considered in justifying department staffing.
2. Define how clinical dietitian behavior can positively and negatively impact how the hospital client makes decisions for the food service department.
3. Determine approaches to assist the clinical dietitians in seeing the big picture.

Case Narrative

Charting in the medical record varies by state licensure law. For example, Maryland licensure law prohibits nonlicensed dietitians or nutritionists from completing a nutrition assessment unless they are under the direct supervision of a licensed dietitian or nutritionist. The following scenario is based on this situation.

Background

This case takes place in a 500-bed skilled nursing facility associated with and physically adjacent to a Veterans Administration (VA) medical center. The nursing facility has four diet technicians (two full-time and two part-time) and two dietitians. There are two diet technicians scheduled every day, and the dietitians work Monday through Friday and are on call over the weekends. The dietitians have home access to the hospital computer system. This allows them to review a patient's laboratory data at any time if needed. The job responsibilities of the dietetic technicians are as follows:

1. Print reports from the computer including a daily list of all residents by unit with diet orders, between meal nourishments by unit, resident likes and dislikes by unit, resident beverage selections by unit, and a daily list of residents with diet orders for no food by mouth (NPO), clear or full liquids, or tube feeding by 7:00 A.M.
2. Print a list of the residents due for MDS* Day 5, 14, 30, and 60-day assessments over the next few days.
3. Review the monthly and quarterly calendars to identify any long-term care residents who need to be assessed that day.
4. Collect data on nutrition assessment forms for newly admitted residents and collect all data for quarterly assessments.
5. Make meal rounds for two meals (early technician does breakfast and lunch; late technician does lunch and dinner) so that all units are visited at least once a day. Information on intake is recorded on a resident list by room number. Any issues identified are brought to the dietitians during 1 P.M. daily meeting.
6. Attend care plan meetings on long-term care units.
7. Fill out quarterly assessment form on all stable, long-term patients, which the dietitian reviews and then countersigns. Technicians do not do quarterly reviews on tube feeders, patients on parenteral nutrition (usually only 1 or 2 patients), or initial follow-up on anyone with significant weight loss.

The job responsibilities of the dietitians are as follows:

1. Review technician prioritization each morning and countersign quarterly assessments, which are then put in the medical record (chart).
2. Complete required assessments of residents on skilled units. Reassign patients found to be low functioning to the technicians for follow-up.
3. Complete initial evaluation and care plan on all long-term residents with weight loss, low albumins, or new breakdown. Complete monthly evaluations on tube feeders.
4. On weekends, review computer information from 9 A.M. to 10 A.M. daily to determine any changes necessary in TPN or high-risk tube feedings; any changes are called in to nursing units. Dietitians accrue one hour of comp time for every hour spent on weekends.

---

*MDS stands for *minimum data set*. This is a detailed assessment form that addresses several aspects of a patient's health and well-being, including nutritional status and dietary intake. Federal regulations require that this form be filled out at regular intervals during a patient's stay in a long-term care facility and submitted by computer.

History and Type of Staffing

Originally the skilled nursing facility had 3½ dietitians with an average cost of $20 per hour (excluding benefits). As turnover occurred, the skilled nursing facility hired graduates of four-year dietetic programs as full-time technicians and third- and fourth-year dietetic students as part-time technicians. The technicians were paid an average of $10 per hour (excluding benefits), and only full-time employees were eligible for benefits. Two 8-hour technicians work Monday through Friday. On weekends one 8-hour technician and one 4-hour technician work due to the lower census count. With the new system there has been reduced turnover in full-time positions, and the administration has been pleased with the reduced costs of recruiting, the reduced cost of agency dietitians, and the resulting improvement in patient care.

Current Challenges

Mrs. Chang is the chief dietitian at the skilled nursing facility. She was recently visited by the new administrator in charge of food and environmental services. He told her that he believes the dietary department has too many staff dietitians and technicians. When Mrs. Chang asked why he felt this way, he stated that at his previous position, a medical center with a larger number of patients, there were fewer dietetic technicians and dietitians. He went on to tell Mrs. Chang that he wanted a written justification for existing staffing levels within the next 72 hours.

   Mrs. Chang was just recuperating from the visit by the hospital administrator when the dietetic technicians came to her with a concern of their own. They complained that the weights of many patients on the long-term care unit are not being measured and recorded by the nursing staff. In fact, one of the nurses told them that they just guess at the weights and actually do not weigh patients. Mrs. Chang was wishing she could start this day over!

Questions

1. How would you handle the request from the new administrator for a written justification of the current staffing levels for dietitians and dietetic technicians?

2. How would you deal with the concerns of the dietetic technicians regarding the lack of correct information on patients' weights? Remember that measurement and recording of weights is a nursing responsibility but is necessary for nutritional assessment of any resident.

Marketing Outpatient Nutrition Counseling

Objectives

At the completion of this case study, students should be able to:

1. Identify creative ways to educate the medical staff on services provided by an outpatient dietitian.
2. Identify potential resources to assist in the marketing of outpatient nutrition services.

Case Narrative

Outpatient nutrition counseling is offered by registered, licensed dietitians for individuals wanting to improve their health through better nutrition. Registered dietitians are experts in nutrition counseling. They provide accurate and current nutrition information and teach patients how to apply it in their lives, and they also work closely with physicians by providing patient reports. Dietary programs can be designed on an individual basis to meet each patient's personal needs. Some common reasons patients may visit a registered dietitian are nutrition for pregnancy, gestational diabetes, pediatric nutrition, weight loss or gain, diabetes, hypoglycemia, hypertension, heart disease, and kidney failure. While it is possible for patients to refer themselves to a dietitian, outpatient nutrition clinics depend on physician referrals for the majority of their appointments.

At Fairhaven Medical Center, the dietitian staff noticed a declining number of referrals for outpatient nutrition counseling in 1999. They did a complete evaluation of the outpatient program, surveyed patients receiving the service, and determined the need to adjust the way nutrition information was presented to the patients. A new dietitian with an extensive background in nutrition counseling was hired, and all of the Center physicians were made aware of the change via the monthly physician newsletter. The next strategy was to increase physician awareness of the programs offered by our outpatient dietitian.

With the help of a marketing representative from the Center and a good brainstorming session, several good ideas were produced regarding ways to reach the physicians. After reviewing the Center's physician directory, the dietitians produced a list of doctors most likely to refer patients based on the nature of their medical specialty. Marketing efforts were targeted toward these physicians. The marketing representative contacted each of the specified physician offices and requested five-minute appointments with the physician, outpatient dietitian, and marketing representative. Some physicians agreed to the appointments, while others did not.

A meeting was convened between the dietitian staff and the marketing representative. The team wanted to come up with a creative way to educate physicians who were new to the outpatient dietitian services while thanking physicians who were currently referring patients to our outpatient dietitian. After brainstorming for some time, we put a formal plan into place.

Questions

1. What types of services does an outpatient dietitian provide?
2. What are some ways to increase physician awareness of the services provided by a registered dietitian? List two creative ways that outpatient nutrition counseling can be marketed to physicians.
3. How might you thank those physicians who do use the service?

Inappropriate Employee Self-Termination

Objectives

At the completion of this case study, students should be able to:

1. Identify the problems and issues encountered when giving inadequate notice.
2. Define what is currently considered proper notice.
3. List several situations in which one could leave a job without proper notice.

Case Narrative

SI, a registered dietitian (RD) who was approximately one year out of his internship, worked in a 300-bed hospital with three other registered dietitians. The nutrition department was managed by a national contract food service company, and all dietitians were employed by the company. SI's clinical nutrition manager (CNM), also an RD, worked hard with SI to help him pass the registration examination, take an early paid vacation, and develop his goals for growth and promotion. In addition, the contract company had paid all moving expenses for SI and his roommate. During his orientation, SI was given the facility policies and procedures, which explained that two weeks' notice was expected with any resignation of professional staff. He had told the CNM and others in the company that he was satisfied with his job and particularly enjoyed training dietetic interns for a local college.

SI had some personal issues. His live-in roommate wanted him to make more money so she could quit her job and go to college full-time. He also wanted to learn how to work as a dietitian in long-term care, since his internship had included no

107

rotations in long-term care. Long-term care experience was not necessary for his employment in the hospital.

Shortly after reaching his one-year mark of employment at the facility, SI gave his CNM his resignation with nine days' notice. SI told his CNM that he had been offered a position as a regional manager for a small private nursing home chain; he would oversee the dietitians in all of the nursing homes in the chain. SI was made aware that he was not leaving with proper notice. He said he was taking the job because it paid more money. He understood that the CNM and the contract company would not be allowed to provide a reference for him since he had given such short notice. Despite requests to leave with proper notice, SI left the facility after nine workdays.

Questions

1. What short-term and long-term issues or problems has SI created for himself by his choice in resigning?
2. How much notice is really necessary for giving proper notice?
3. Are there any circumstances in which giving less than proper notice would be considered appropriate?
4. Do you think SI is adequately trained for the regional manager position? What might SI do to maximize his chances of success in this new job?

Cases in Financial Management

BUDGET PLANNING TO IMPROVE THE BOTTOM LINE

MEALS PER LABOR HOUR: INTERPRETING THE DATA

PRODUCTIVITY MEASURES EXERCISE

Budget Planning to Improve the Bottom Line

Objectives

At the completion of this case study, students should be able to:

1. Recognize the ongoing challenges of annual budget preparation and financial performance monitoring.
2. Describe the difference between top-line and bottom-line growth.
3. Recognize the benefits of benchmarking with peer businesses.

Case Narrative

Colleen is the director of a department that has a budget that runs in the millions of dollars. This department is in a healthcare setting, so the bottom line (net profit margin) is negative since patient food services are a cost center without any significant associated revenue. The reason for this is that patient food service is considered to be part of the room charge.

Colleen's calendar indicates that budget planning will begin soon for the next fiscal year. The executive that she reports to has indicated that with continued increases in labor costs, the budget must be based upon a 0 percent increase in non-labor costs. In addition, the goal is to improve the bottom line by increasing revenue, if possible.

An effective method to improve financial planning is to benchmark departmental costs and statistical data against other, similar-sized organizations. Benchmarking provides opportunities to enhance revenue, control costs, and improve overall financial performance. Comparisons of departmental revenue, costs, and statistical data assist all participants in the establishment of future best practices.

111

It is important to understand the difference between top-line growth and bottom-line growth. Top-line growth is an increase in revenue independent of increases or decreases in expenses. Bottom-line growth is an improvement of the difference between revenue (top-line sales) and expenses from one accounting period to another (month-to-month and year-to-year). Bottom-line equals net income or net margin.

The spreadsheet represents cost and statistical information to be used and reviewed in the benchmark operations. Uniformity is critical for effective analysis. This spreadsheet is designed to capture information for a twelve-month period. Actual data from the most recently completed fiscal year or projected actual data from the current fiscal year are used.

Although most cost/statistical categories are self-explanatory, the categories described in Table 1 may require further explanation:

Some questions to ask during benchmark analysis include:

- Where are the opportunities to improve the bottom line; that is, cause it to be less negative?
- How can a department director determine whether the current revenues and expenses are realistic for this type of business?
- Can a department director increase his or her top-line growth? How?
- How can a department director decrease some of the expense lines?

The workbook for this case includes two spreadsheets, Figures 1 and 2. Figure 1 outlines the characteristics of each organization. Figure 2 includes the financial information for each organization.

Questions

Upon completion of the information from the participating businesses, Colleen needs to analyze the differences.

Table 1   Definitions of Cost/Statistical Categories

Category	Description
Revenue	All sales income (not credits) received from various operations such as retail, vending, catering, convenience stores, and client nutrition consulting.
Food Cost	All food costs charged to the department.
Payroll	All payroll costs charged to the department including outside temporary labor. Do not include benefits, taxes, etc., in this category. Typically salary scales will be comparable between peer businesses; however, the benefit package may differ significantly.
Direct Cost	All direct expenses such as paper, plastic, cleaning supplies, insurance, meeting expenses, phone service, maintenance and repairs, and general supply requisition charges.

Characteristics of Each Organization

	Colleen's ORG	ORG A	ORG B	ORG C
Points of Service				
Patients	Yes, same building	Yes, same building	Yes, same building	Yes, same building
Cafeterias	2 Cafés	2 Cafés	1 Café	1 Café
Vending	Receives commission	Receives commission	Does own vending	No income
Catering (cash)	No	Yes	Yes	No
Coffee kiosk in lobby	No	Yes	No	No
Meals on wheels, day care centers	No	No	Yes	No
Outpatient nutrition consultation	No	No	Yes	No
Food Purchasing	Purchasing group	Purchasing group	Purchasing group	Purchasing group
Food Production System	Cook serve	Cook serve	Cook serve	Cook serve
Weekly Menu Planning Focus	Medium	Medium	High	Medium
Department Payroll				
Regional renal dialysis center	Yes	No	No	No
Provide all environmental service needs for department	Yes	No	No	No
Provide night (3rd shift) food service	Yes	Yes	No	No
Provide host/hostess program for patients	Yes	Yes	No	No
Direct Costs				
Serviceware for patients	China	China	China	China
Serviceware for staff and visitors	China	Disposables	China	China
Statistics				
Total Meals	551,695	650,728	479,647	400,722
Café meal factors	$6.22	$5.25	$6.07	$5.00
Beds	490	236	400	254
	Tertiary care hospital	Full service hospital	Full service hospital	Tertiary care hospital
Patient days (less newborns)	79,321	87,600	66,429	59,452

Figure 1   Food and Nutrition Services Benchmarking: Characteristics

	Colleen's ORG	ORG A	ORG B	ORG C
Revenue:				
Cafeteria sales	$1,295,651	$1,100,000	$918,168	$690,899
Vending sales	$68,088	$0	$211,658	$0
Catering (cash)	$11,571	$364,000	$9,048	$0
Misc. rev.-meals on wheels, day care centers	$0	$0	$56,540	$0
Outpatient nutrition consultation			$195,000	
Total Retail Revenue	**$1,375,310**	**$1,464,000**	**$1,390,414**	**$690,899**
Expenses:				
Total food cost	$1,328,737	$1,643,650	$1,112,783	$1,045,896
Payroll cost - salaries and wages	$2,202,999	$2,843,206	$1,529,426	$1,484,352
Direct costs - minus depreciation	$487,975	$766,663	$592,707	$378,124
Total Expenses (food, labor, direct)	**$4,019,711**	**$5,253,519**	**$3,234,916**	**$2,908,372**
Special function (credit)	($297,958)	$0	($213,874)	($176,384)
Floor stock (credit)	($99,290)	($216,000)	($52,308)	($54,749)
Misc. (credit)	($164,606)	($458,000)	$0	($44,245)
Total (credits)	**($561,854)**	**($674,000)**	**($266,182)**	**($275,378)**
Total Adjusted Expenses	**$3,457,857**	**$4,579,519**	**$2,968,734**	**$2,632,994**
Statistics				
Revenue % of Adj. Expenses	39.8%	32.0%	46.8%	26.2%
Total FTEs Actual	88.6	84.4	61.4	58.7
FTE Normalization-differences relative to other organizations	64.7	84.4	61.4	58.7
Renal RDs	3.0			
Janitors/PM driver	3.1			
Night service	1.9			

Clinic café				2.5
Patient nutrition assistants				12.2
Vacuuming of dining rooms				1.2
Average hourly rate for client FTE	$10.85	$10.42	$16.20	$10.70
Total meals	400,722	479,647	650,728	551,695
Food Cost per Meal-Actual	**$2.61**	**$2.32**	**$2.53**	**$2.41**
Café meal factors	$5.00	$6.07	$5.25	$6.22
Patient days (less newborns)	59,452	66,429	87,600	79,321
Total NET Adj Expenses per Patient Day	**$44.29**	**$44.69**	**$52.28**	**$43.59**
Food Expense per Patient Day	**$17.59**	**$17.50**	**$18.76**	**$16.75**
Labor Expense per Patient Day	**$24.97**	**$23.02**	**$32.46**	**$27.77**
Direct Expense per Patient Day	**$6.36**	**$8.92**	**$8.75**	**$6.15**

Figure 2   Food and Nutrition Services Benchmarking: Financial Information

Revenue/Sales

1. Do any of the benchmark businesses have higher sales or income than Colleen's business? What are the differences? Can Colleen initiate additional products or services to increase her own top-line sales?

Payroll Costs and Full-Time Equivalents

2. Do any of the benchmark businesses have lower labor hours than Colleen's business? Can Colleen implement systems or processes that would reduce the overall labor-hour requirements and as a result lower her payroll costs?

Non-Labor Expenses

3. Do any of the benchmark businesses have lower expenses in any of the major categories of food or supplies? What purchasing practices can Colleen implement to lower her food and supply costs—group purchasing, prime vendor, or other strategy? What utilization practices can Colleen implement to lower food and supply costs—menu planning, recipe standardization, portion control, or other strategy?

Meals per Labor Hour

Interpreting the Data

Objectives

At the completion of this case study, students should be able to:

1. Describe how meals per labor hour is calculated.
2. Identify the information needed to calculate meals per labor hour data.
3. Analyze meals per labor hour data and explain the reasons for differences in meals per labor hour between facilities.
4. Describe at least one benefit of being well networked and involved in one's professional association.

Case Narrative

Part One

Mira is the director of food and nutrition services at Platt Regional Medical Center in a medium-sized hospital in the Mid-Atlantic Region of the United States. The food and nutrition department produces and serves approximately 725 patient meals and 850 cafeteria meals per day. It also sends approximately 150 nourishments to patients each day and averages 30 catered meals per day. The dietary department also stocks all the vending machines in the facility.

Mira reports directly to Jack Platt, a hospital administrator who also oversees environmental services and building maintenance. Jack recently talked to a colleague who oversees food services at Mercy Medical Center, a neighboring hospital. The colleague told Jack that the dietary department averages 4.5 meals per labor hour. Jack checked the data sent to him by Mira and found that her department

117

Table 1 Area Medical Centers and Their Meals per Labor Hour

Medical Center	Number of Meals per Labor Hour
Mercy Medical Center	4.5
Watkins County Regional Medical Center	4.1
Union County Hospital	3.8
Platt Regional Medical Center (Mira's department)	3.5

averaged only 3.5 meals per labor hour. Puzzled, he called a few other colleagues at neighboring hospitals and collected the information presented in Table 1.

Alarmed, Jack called Mira to his office. When she arrived, he asked her to sit down and presented the data to her. She studied it for a minute and then asked Jack to give her a week to respond to his concerns. When Mira returned to her office, she decided she needed to collect some information about the other facilities before she addressed the issue with Jack.

Questions

1. How is meals per labor hour traditionally calculated?
2. What information would you want to collect about the food service departments in each of these hospitals?
3. How might you obtain this information?

Part Two

Luckily, Mira was very active in her professional association and thus knew dietitians and food service managers at both Mercy Medical Center and Union County Hospital. She called them and gathered the information she needed. One of her friends at Mercy also had a contact at Watkins Medical Center and put her in touch with a food service manager who could give her the needed information for his facility. She put together the information shown in Table 2.

Mira then sat down to consider the information in the table in front of her. She immediately wished she had asked a few more questions about the facilities but decided to formulate a response given the data available.

Questions

1. How many meals per person per day is Mira serving? Why is it not three meals per day as might initially be expected?
2. What other information should Mira have obtained?

Table 2   Information Collected on Area Medical Centers

Medical Center	Information
Mercy Medical Center	• Average census: 70 patients • Small employee cafeteria • Ready-serve system where 90 percent of hot food is purchased frozen and reheated for service • Minimal catering • Vending done by contractor
Watkins County Regional Medical Center	• Average census: 650 patients • Large employee cafeteria • Considerable catering • Sends meals to nursing home • Vending machines stocked by the food service department
Union County Hospital	• Average census: 240 patients • Medium-sized cafeteria • Minimal catering • Vending done by a contractor
Platt Regional Medical Center (Mira's department)	• Average census: 265 patients • Medium-sized cafeteria • Minimal catering • Vending machines stocked by the food service department

3. Looking at Table 2, what are some reasonable explanations for why Mira's meals per labor hour figure is lower than these other facilities?

4. Mira calculates her meals per labor hour by dividing total meals by total labor hours. She determines her total meals served by taking a count of how many patient meals are served and adding in the number of cafeteria and catering meals served. Cafeteria meals are determined by taking total sales and dividing by an average cost for a typical meal ($2.45). Catering meals are determined similarly, but with a different average check cost. Mira decides to call the other three facilities again and ask them how they calculate their meals per labor hour. What might she find out? Would a difference in calculation of meals per labor hour help explain some of the variation in the numbers in Table 1? If so, how?

Productivity Measures Exercise

Objectives

At the completion of this case study, students should be able to:

1. Correctly calculate numbers of meals and revenue from raw numbers typically received in a food service operation.
2. Correctly calculate productivity formulas.
3. Determine level of productivity from a given scenario.
4. Interpret findings of productivity measures and make recommendations.

Case Narrative

St. John's Medical Center is a not-for-profit acute care facility licensed for one hundred beds. It is located in a northwestern town with a population base of 80,000. The average census is 52, of which 20 percent are NPO (no food by mouth) at any given time. In addition to traditional patient tray service, an average of seventy-two nourishments are prepared and delivered on a daily basis. The meal equivalent for patient meals is valued at $6.50 per meal. Six nourishments are equal in value to one patient tray.

St. John's also has a cafeteria and catering services. The cafeteria serves 100 breakfasts, 250 lunches, and 75 dinners per day on average. Cafeteria sales average $1,500.00 per day. Catering services vary depending upon the month and day of the week and services required. The average monthly revenue is $3,000.00 with approximately five hundred meals per month ($6.00 meal equivalent) being served.

Finally, St. John's Medical Center has won the bid for providing home delivered meals to the surrounding communities. They provide one hundred meals, seven days a week and are reimbursed at a rate of $5.00 per meal from the local community action agency which oversees the program.

Raw food costs equal 38 percent of total revenue. Labor hours run 152 per day at an average salary of $7.75 per hour plus 30 percent for benefits for all employees (both full- and part-time).

Questions

1. Calculate the following from the above information:
   a. FTEs (full-time equivalents)
   b. Meals per labor hour
   c. Labor cost per meal served
   d. Percent labor of total revenue
   e. Productivity based upon industry standards (be sure to categorize)
2. Summarize the productivity of the staff. How does it compare to published staffing indices? Is productivity adequate? If not, how might it be improved?
3. What are some legitimate reasons for differing productivity rates among food service operations?

Resources

Spears, M. C. and M. Gregoire, 2004. *Foodservice Organizations: A Managerial and Systems Approach,* 5th ed. Upper Saddle River, NJ: Prentice Hall.

Lieux, E. M. and P. K. Luoto, 2001. *Exploring Quantity Food Production and Service through Problems,* 2nd ed. Upper Saddle River, NJ: Prentice Hall.

Cases Rated by Degree of Difficulty

**(1 = fairly simple or easy,
3 = fairly complex or difficult)**

Introduction

Cases as Teaching Tools

Cases in Menu Management

Cases in Purchasing

Cases in Food Production

Cases in Service

Cases in Safety and Sanitation

Cases in Management of Food Services

Cases in Nutrition Management

Cases in Financial Management